MW01502616

Radial and Astigmatic Keratotomy

The American System of Precise, Predictable Refractive Surgery

Radial and Astigmatic Keratotomy

The American System of Precise, Predictable Refractive Surgery

Spencer P. Thornton, MD, FACS

Foreword by Professor S.N. Fyodorov, MD

SLACK Incorporated, 6900 Grove Road, Thorofare, NJ 08086-9447

Managing Editor: Amy E. Drummond
Cover Design: Linda Baker
Publisher: John H. Bond
Project Editor: Debra L. Clarke

The procedures and practices described in this book should be implemented in a manner consistent with the professional standards set for the circumstances that apply in each specific situation. Every effort has been made to confirm the accuracy of the information presented and to correctly relate generally accepted practices. The authors, editor, and publisher cannot accept responsibility for errors or exclusions or for the outcome of the application of the material presented herein. There is no expressed or implied warranty of this book or information imparted by it.

Care has been taken to ensure that drug selection and dosages are in accordance with currently accepted/recommended practice. Due to continuing research, changes in government policy and regulations, and various effects of drug reactions and interactions, it is recommended that the reader carefully review all materials and literature provided for each drug, especially those that are new or not frequently used.

Thornton, Spencer P.
Radial and astigmatic keratotomy: the American system/Spencer P. Thornton
  p. cm.
  Includes bibliographical references and index.
  ISBN 1-55642-238-5
  1. Eye--Refractive errors--Surgery. 2. Keratotomy, Radial. 3. Cornea--Surgery.
  I. Title. [DNLM: 1. Astigmatism--surgery. 2. Keratotomy, Radial--methods.
  WW 310 T514r 1994]
  RE336.T48 1994
  617.7'55--dc20
  DNLM/DLC   94-4186
                                           CIP

Printed in the United States of America

Published by: SLACK Incorporated
                6900 Grove Road
                Thorofare, NJ 08086-9447

Last digit is print number: 10   9   8   7   6   5   4   3   2   1

Dedication

To Ginnie, my beloved wife and very best friend.
Without her patience and support, this book would not have been written.

Contents

Foreword

For about 20 years the method of radial keratotomy has been used for the surgical correction of myopia and astigmatism. A great number of clinical investigations that were carried out during this period proved the high efficiency and safety of this technology, and many people received the opportunity to see this beautiful world without any sophisticated optical devices.

In the beginning many surgeons rejected keratotomy, being afraid of putting it into practice, and some of them openly struggled against it. But finally common sense won, and radial keratotomy received the world recognition it deserved.

Although there are many different methods of myopia correction, such as keratomileusis, excimer laser and posterior chamber negative power lens implantation, refractive keratotomy is taking a stable position in refractive surgery, remaining the only sure method of myopic astigmatism correction.

Dr. Spencer Thornton was one of the first surgeons who applied radial and astigmatic keratotomy in the USA. The results proved to be brilliant. Nowadays the works of Spencer Thornton concerning the application of keratotomy in cases of myopia and astigmatism are well known all over the world, and they have played a great role in the development of radial and astigmatic keratotomy in and outside the USA.

As an experienced surgeon known all over the world, Spencer Thornton has contributed much to the training of qualified personnel in refractive surgery. The surgeons use the instruments suggested by Dr. Thornton, and use his nomograms for keratotomy calculation.

This book is a summary of long practical experience and theoretical investigations of Spencer Thornton. This makes it very useful from the practical point of view for surgeons eager to master the methods of radial and astigmatic keratotomy.

S.N. Fyodorov, MD
Professor, Director
Moscow Research Institute of Eye Microsurgery

Acknowledgments

In a work of this type there are a number of individuals who should be acknowledged for their contributions. First I wish to acknowledge the special contributions of my staff, Jean Robertson, Celeste Thompson and Frances Parker, who provide an environment that is supportive of the demands of book authorship while maintaining a busy clinical practice. Jean Robertson, RN, COT, in addition to her numerous professional responsibilities, assisted in preparing the text, and developed the system of forms and patient education materials used in our practice found in Appendix C. Celeste Thompson typed and retyped much of the original manuscript with a dedication that is rare, adding the burden of this book to her already heavy responsibilities as secretary and office manager.

I'm grateful to Donald R. Sanders, MD, PhD, for his constant encouragement and valuable advice, and the staff of the Center for Clinical Research for data analysis both in the chapters on Astigmatic Keratotomy results and Corneal Topography. Chuck Hess and Michelle Glossip of Storz Instrument Company and Doug Mastel of Mastel Designs provided several of the instrument pictures in Chapter 5, and Doug Mastel provided valuable information on diamond blade design. Keith Yeisley, president of Metico, gave inspiration and help in a number of ways. Dr. Gerald Marinoff and the G and G Medical Instrument Company provided valuable assistance in instrument inspection.

This book is the outgrowth of years of investigation, clinical application and course presentations. This didn't occur in a vacuum. The International Society of Refractive Keratoplasty (ISRK) provided the forum to present new and controversial ideas through its symposia and its Journal, and the American Society of Cataract and Refractive Surgery (ASCRS) provided me the opportunity to present these ideas in Society sponsored courses beginning in 1985, with Drs. David Davis, Jim Hays, Skip Nichamin, Johnny Gayton, Harold Stein, John Corboy and other colleagues joining me as faculty, and through its *Journal of Cataract and Refractive Surgery*.

I thank SLACK Publisher John Bond and Editor Amy Drummond who insisted that this book be published, and Debra Clarke and the staff at SLACK who guided the organization of the book and illustrations to a finished product in record time.

I want to acknowledge the numerous sources of information that contributed to the system which is the backbone of this book. Because many of these sources are not specifically referred to in the text, they are listed in Appendix E as Recommended Reading.

Finally I wish to acknowledge my debt of gratitude to the numerous colleagues who have used the material in this book, originally presented in my courses, and encouraged me to put it in book form.

About the Author

Dr. Thornton earned his MD from the Bowman Gray School of Medicine at Wake Forest University, and completed his residency in ophthalmology at Vanderbilt University School of Medicine.

He is certified by the American Board of Ophthalmology, Fellow of the American Academy of Ophthalmology, Fellow of the American College of Surgeons, a member of the Board of Directors of the American College of Eye Surgeons, and Secretary of the International Refractive Surgery Club. He is a member of the Executive Committee of the American Society of Cataract and Refractive Surgery (and is Secretary of that society), and serves as Chairman of the International Committee on Standards and Quality Control for Ophthalmic Instruments and Devices.

His professional activities include: member of the Editorial Board of *Refractive and Corneal Surgery*, member of the Editorial Board of the *Video Journal of Ophthalmology*, member of the Editorial Board of *Ocular Surgery News*, contributing editor to *Ophthalmic Practice* (Canada), and Associate Editor of the *Journal of Cataract and Refractive Surgery*.

Dr. Thornton is co-author or contributor to fourteen textbooks on ophthalmic surgery and author of more than 100 published papers on cataract and refractive surgery. He has been adjunct or guest professor in universities in ten countries (U.S., Sweden, Germany, France, South Africa, Switzerland, Greece, Japan, Austria and Canada) and holds honorary life memberships in ophthalmic societies in four countries (Canada, Brazil, Austria and South Africa).

He has lectured in twenty-seven countries: U.S., Canada, Argentina, Brazil, Colombia, Mexico, Venezuela, Sweden, Denmark, England, Russia, France, Germany, Austria, Switzerland, Spain, Hungary, Ireland, Scotland, Italy, Greece, South Africa, Australia, New Zealand, China, Japan and Thailand.

Dr. Thornton is a member of the Board of Visitors of Baylor University and Director of the Thornton Eye Surgery Center in Nashville, Tennessee.

Introduction

Refractive surgery is finding its way into the practices of an increasing number of ophthalmic surgeons around the world, and for good reason. Radial keratotomy and astigmatic keratotomy have been shown to be safe and effective tools with which to achieve emmetropia in the majority of the myopic and astigmatic population and with cataract patients who have undergone intraocular lens implantation.

Several hundred thousand radial keratotomy procedures have been performed in the United States by approximately 10% of the ophthalmologists. In the rest of the world fewer than 3% of the ophthalmologists perform the procedure, but these numbers are increasing as more and more ophthalmologists are participating in basic and advanced refractive surgery courses.

Radial keratotomy was over-promoted in the early years after its introduction to America in 1978, leading to wide criticism of the procedure and its proponents. But, thanks to a number of conservative surgeons who, individually and in coordinated efforts, persisted in a careful investigative approach, the procedures gradually gained acceptance and are now being added to the armamentarium of most progressive ophthalmologists.

In this book I've made every effort to bring you the most dependable system of refractive surgery available. It is based on material that was developed over a period of fifteen years of experience with incisional refractive surgery, and has been revised and updated to include information derived from thousands of cases done by many surgeons using these nomograms.

In developing the American system of precise and predictable radial keratotomy and astigmatic keratotomy I have learned from and been encouraged by many excellent surgeons, all of whom unselfishly shared their ideas and suggestions, some testing my nomograms, others suggesting modifications and new applications, others giving valuable advice. To these I owe much. Among these are Leo Bores, Slava Fyodorov, Dennis Shepard, Don Sanders, Al Neumann, Bob Fenzl, Jim Hays, David Davis, John Corboy, Dick Lindstrom, George Waring, Marguerite McDonald, Lee Nordan, Johnny Gayton and others. And the list continues to grow.

I was among the first Americans to become involved in radial keratotomy and in 1979 performed my first few cases of RK and AK—and seeing what joy it brought to those who benefited from it, I decided to add it to cataract surgery as my chief interest. When, in the early 1980s RK came under attack by some in the academic community, I never stopped doing it, and never stopped teaching it to those colleagues who, like me, wanted to add to the quality of vision of their patients by the elimination of surgically-correctable errors.

My first nomograms for myopia and astigmatism were published in 1982 and have been refined and modified several times over the years to take advantage of new information and improved instrumentation which has contributed to greater precision and greater predictability. But, as you'll discover in comparing the early nomograms with those in this book, the modifications have been few and the basic principles have remained the same.

My prime concern for the surgeon learning radial and astigmatic keratotomy is that he be given a nomogram for surgical planning which is reasonable, straightforward and easily understood, so that he can get an overall feeling of how the operation works without being limited to a simplistic mathematical grid which gives an inaccurate projection as to the accuracy of the operation. It is my hope that the principles outlined in this book will enable you to achieve a level of success that will bring both satisfaction and pleasure in your refractive surgery practice.

Surgery for myopia and astigmatism should be tailored to the patient, not the patient to the surgery. The nomogram and its modifiers should be carefully followed. With care and attention to proper surgical planning, your results will be more accurate and bring a great deal of pleasure to you and your patients. I wish you well in your quest.

Spencer P. Thornton, MD, FACS

1

History of Radial and Astigmatic Keratotomy

Nearsighted people have sought ways to improve their distance vision and rid themselves of eyeglasses for centuries. Ancient Chinese scholars are said to have slept with sandbags on their eyes to flatten their corneas, and medical and surgical attempts at reducing myopia have challenged some of the great minds of history.

In 1898, Dr. L. J. Lans, of Leiden, the Netherlands, published the results of experiments with rabbits in treating astigmatism with keratectomy, keratotomy and thermokeratoplasty.[1] After studying the effect of corneal incisions, he stated three basic principles of keratotomy.

1. The cornea flattens in the meridian of the incision.

2. Some of the effect is lost as shallow incisions heal.

3. Incisions must penetrate through most of the cornea to obtain a lasting effect.

In 1933, Professor Tsutomu Sato observed a patient with keratoconus who developed an acute break in Descemet's membrane followed by spontaneous healing, flattening of the cornea, and improvement of vision. Another similar observation in 1936 led him to conclude that deliberately made incisions in the corneal endothelium would be beneficial in the treatment of keratoconus and astigmatism.[2]

In cooperation with Dr. Koichiro Akiyama, Dr. Sato performed extensive laboratory experiments with animals which led to the identification of the two main methods of modifying corneal curvature, radial and transverse incisions. He proposed two basic patterns: posterior transverse incisions in the steep axis for mild astigmatism and posterior transverse incisions and radial incisions in the steep axis for more severe myopia and astigmatism.

The result of the Sato experiments was a procedure that involved some forty to forty-five radial incisions through Descemet's membrane posteriorly and an additional forty or so through the anterior surface of the cornea, using a clear optical zone of about 5mm.

In thirty-two cases followed up to four months he reported a mean reduction of refractive myopia of 2.80D, with a range of 1.50 to 7.00D. He observed that the deeper cuts and the posterior cuts produced the greatest flattening, and in 1953 reported that, "no detrimental effects from this procedure have been observed."[3]

After many years of observation, investigators from Juntendo University in Tokyo found that about 86% of eyes followed for twenty-five to thirty years developed bullous keratopathy an average of twenty years after surgery, and researchers found that despite subepithelial edema and disruption and destruction of endothelium, there was enough reserve to maintain corneal clarity in most eyes for a decade or two before it failed.[4]

Because of the honesty and forthrightness of the Japanese researchers in reporting the failures of the Sato procedures, radial keratotomy was abandoned for some ten to fifteen years. Then in the early 1970s Yenaliev, Durnev and Fyodorov, aware of the corneal edema and decompensation that resulted from Sato's posterior incisions, began studying anterior radial corneal incisions for myopia. In 1974, Dr. Svyatoslav N. Fyodorov began radial keratotomy surgery in humans and over the next few years made a series of observations:[5]

1. Sixteen incisions gave almost the same results as did 20, 24 and 32 incisions.

2. Larger diameter corneas produced more flattening than smaller corneas.

3. Steeper corneas gave greater effect than flatter corneas.

4. Smaller diameters of the central clear zone gave a greater reduction in myopia.

5. Age affected the result, with a higher "coefficient of scleral rigidity" with age, increasing the reduction of myopia.

6. The surgeon's individual technique determined the correlation of the theoretical result with the actual result.

Radial keratotomy and astigmatic keratotomy were introduced to the United States by Dr. Fyodorov and Dr. Leo Bores in 1978. Initially, the procedure and its proponents were widely criticized. But, thanks to a number of conservative surgeons who, individually and in coordinated efforts, persisted in a careful investigative approach, the procedures gradually gained acceptance, and over the next several years a number of studies verified the relative safety and efficacy of incisional keratotomy for the correction of myopia and astigmatism, and today the progressive ophthalmologist has added corneal relaxing incisions (CRIs) to his or her surgical armamentarium for all types of myopia and astigmatism.

Refractive surgery for congenital and surgically induced astigmatism is now recognized as a natural result of recent developments in technology and instrumentation, with new diamond micrometer knives, accurate to the hundredth of a millimeter, and corneal topography devices offering a means of planning and following corneal surgery with unprecedented accuracy. Most important has been a greater understanding of the physiology of the incised cornea and the predictability of effect of altered corneal curvature.

Radial and transverse keratotomy, in the anterior peripheral corneal surface, have been shown to be effective and predictable in reducing myopia and astigmatism. The challenge of the future is unaided emmetropia, and increasing numbers of progressive ophthalmologists are taking basic and advanced courses in RK and AK to learn the techniques of corneal relaxing incisions for the correction of myopia and pre-existing and surgically induced astigmatism.

References

1. Lans LJ: Experimentelle Untersuchungen uber Entstehung von Astigmatissus durch nicht-perforirende Corneawunden. *Albrecht Von Graefes Arch Ophthalmol*, 1898, 45: 117-152.

2. Sato T: Treatment of conical corneal incision of Descemet's membrane. *Acta Soc Ophthalmol Jpn*, 1939, 43: 541.

3. Sato T, Akiyama K, Shibata H: A new surgical approach to myopia. *Am J Ophthalmol*, 1953, 36: 823-829.

4. Akiyama K, Tanaka M, Kanai A, Nakajima A: Problems arising from Sato's radial keratotomy procedure in Japan. *CLAO Journal*, 1984, 10: 179-184.

5. Fyodorov S: Surgical correction of myopia and astigmatism. In: Schachar RA, Levy NS, Schachar L, eds: Keratorefraction: Proceedings of the Keratorefractive Society Meeting. Denison: LAL Publishing, 1980, 141-172.

2

Theory of
Corneal Relaxing Incisions

The Effect of Adding and Removing Tissue

The cornea may be made steeper by removing tissue, as in wedge resection, or by tight suture closure following cataract surgery. As it becomes steeper, the radius of curvature is reduced and the refractive power increased in the steepened meridian. In addition, the keratometric reading is increased in the steepened meridian, reflecting the increased power.

The cornea is made flatter by adding tissue, and an unsutured incision acts as if tissue is added by relaxation of the incised tissue. The radius of curvature is increased, and the keratometric reading and the refractive power are reduced in the flattened meridian. To understand the basis for these effects, we need to look at the theoretical basis for corneal relaxing incisions (CRIs).

The Barrier Principle - Theory and Application

An unsutured incision in the cornea always acts as if tissue is added. The tissue is always "added" or "relaxed" at right angles to the direction of the incision (Figures 2-1a and 2-1b). If the incision is placed radially, its action is transmitted 360° around the circumference of the cornea, provided there are no "barriers."

In the usual RK the first incision (and the second incision, if opposite the first) increases the circumference 360° (Figure 2-2). An incision placed 90°

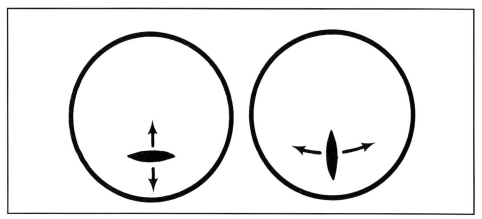

Figure 2-1a. Relaxing incisions act as if tissue is added, and the radius of curvature is increased at right angles to the incision.

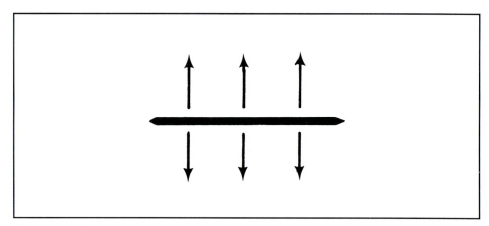

Figure 2-1b. Effect of added tissue is at right angle to the incision.

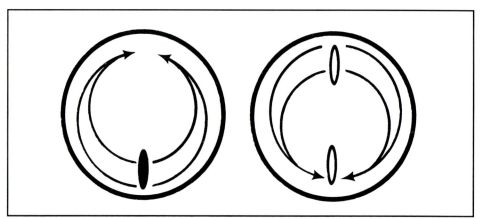

Figure 2-2. Corneal circumference is increased 360° with first two incisions.

away from the first and second incisions (i.e., halfway between the first and second incisions) acts over an area of 180° (i.e., 90° to either side of that incision) until it hits the previously placed incisions which act as a "barrier" (Figure 2-3a). Any subsequently added incisions have their action between adjacent incisions (Figure 2-3b).

Transverse relaxing incisions, whether straight "T" incisions or arcuate incisions, "add tissue" in the meridian across which they are placed (remember, the action produced by an incision is at right angles to the incision). The reason these incisions are so powerful is that their circumferential effect is stopped at the limbus and therefore concentrated by a "limiting barrier," the limbus (Figure 2-4).

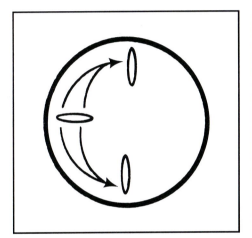

Figure 2-3a.

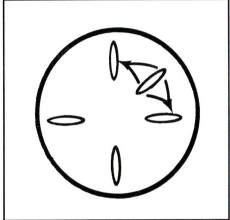

Figure 2-3b.

Figure 2-3. Effect of incisions is primarily in area between previous incisions.

Barrier Tissue

Congruous tissue transmits forces of relaxation or tension uniformly unless impaired in some way. If there is any interference by a "barrier" or discontinuity, this uniformity will be interrupted. Tissues non-congruous to the corneal stroma are the limbus and any scars which may be present in the cornea.

Just as the limbus is a discontinuous tissue to the cornea, the interface of host and donor tissue after penetrating keratoplasty becomes an "artificial limbus," interrupting the continuity and uniformity of the corneal tissue, and will limit the transmission of relaxation of tissue produced by corneal relaxing incisions placed in the donor button to within the donor button itself. Because the area of congruous tissue is smaller, an incision of any given length in a PKP button will have more effect than similar incisions placed in a "virgin" cornea.

Another incision crossing the path of the "effect area" also acts as a barrier. This barrier may impede the effect or enhance it depending of the direction of the

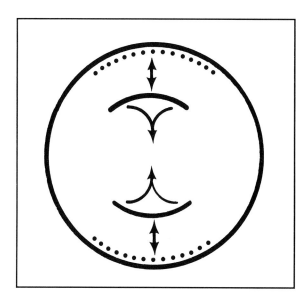

Figure 2-4. Barrier concentrates effect of relaxing incisions.

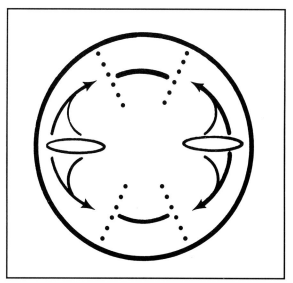

Figure 2-5. Barrier effect of right angles incision.

incision. When that incision is in the same direction (as with additional radial incisions) the effect is enhanced between the radials. When the incision is at right angles to the barrier incision the effect is impeded or restricted, as in the case of combined T incisions and radials (Figure 2-5).

The Limbal Barrier

Since tissue is effectively added with any incision, no matter what its curvature, or lack of curvature, the "added tissue" is at right angles to the incision, and the

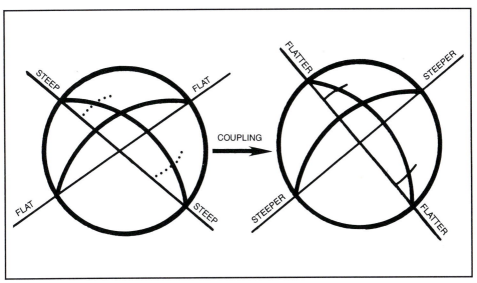

Figure 2-6. Coupling: steepening of the cornea 90° away from transverse relaxing incisions.

effective increase in circumference in the meridian of steep curvature across the corneal dome is limited by the limbus to a "band" across the cornea, the meridional corneal diameter. The limbus thus acts as a "barrier," and confines the effect of the relaxing incisions primarily to the area between the arcuate transverse incisions (see Figure 2-4), much as a megaphone magnifies sound confined within the walls of the megaphone.

Coupling

Whereas radial incisions increase the circumference of the peripheral cornea as they relax tissue around the circumference, *transverse* incisions, if placed parallel to the limbus and concentric to the center of the visual axis, relax only the meridian in which they are placed and do not increase the corneal circumference. If there is no increase in the circumference of the cornea a phenomenon called *coupling* occurs. Coupling is the effect of incisions that relax and flatten the steeper meridian to steepen the flatter meridian 90° away (Figure 2-6).

The coupling effect of transverse incisions is offset or reduced by added radial incisions or transverse incisions which are so long as to become semiradial. All straight lines on a spherical surface are curved (Figure 2-7) and so what appears as a straight corneal incision is actually inversely curved and the ends of the incision are semiradial, and the longer the incision the more radial it becomes (Figure 2-8), reducing any potential coupling.

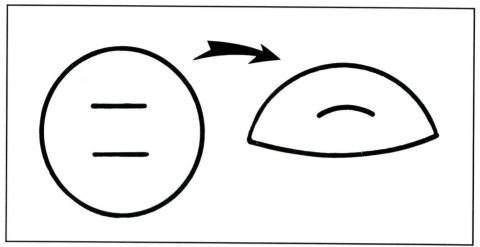

Figure 2-7. Lines on a spherical surface appear straight or curved depending on perspective.

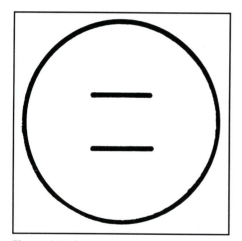

Figure 2-8. Straight transverse incisions are actually inverse arcs and therefore semiradial. The longer the T the more "radial" it becomes.

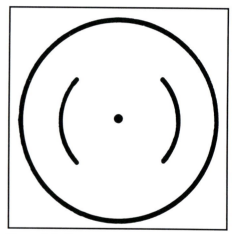

Figure 2-9. True transverse incisions are concentric to the visual axis.

Truly transverse incisions are arcuate incisions which are concentric to the visual axis and parallel to the limbus (Figure 2-9). These incisions have the potential for greater effect because the ends of the incision are at the same distance from the corneal center as the mid portion, that is, are at the same optical zone, and maintain the same corneal depth for the full length of the incision.

Summary

The goal of emmetropia with myopia and astigmatism is now attainable with incisional refractive surgery because of increased understanding of the effect of precisely placed relaxing incisions in the cornea. Even cases with moderate to high errors are responsive to RK and AK when proper case selection and surgical planning are meticulously carried out. Nomograms are available for accurate, predictable radial and astigmatic keratotomy which are as reliable as those for calculation of intraocular lens power, and will be explained in the following chapters.

3

Patient Selection, Work-up and Informed Consent

The decision to undergo an elective refractive surgery procedure is a major and a very personal one. Patients have heard from their friends and read in the press about the dramatic improvement in the quality of life provided by radial keratotomy and astigmatic keratotomy and they have come to you for advice.

You and your staff have the responsibility to educate the patient and to make sure he or she is fully aware of the expected benefits versus the limitations and possible risks of the surgery. No matter how justified the procedure may seem on the basis of physical and refractive qualifications, the decision for surgery must depend on knowledge and understanding of the risks versus the benefits, and that decision must lie with the patient.

It is quite possible to get a 20/20 result and have a dissatisfied patient. Conversely, many RK patients with less than 20/20 vision are thrilled with their results. Patient satisfaction requires that the patient's realistic expectations be met. To achieve this goal, the patient must be thoroughly informed and counseled to accept realistic results, and then the surgery planned and carried out so that the results meet or exceed those expectations.

The patient must be screened to determine if he or she is a good candidate for the surgery, both in terms of refractive needs and general health, as well as to determine his or her psychological suitability (Figure 3-1).

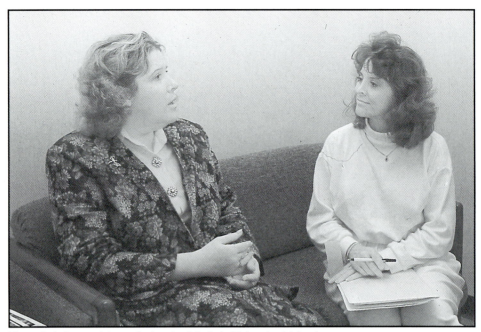

Figure 3-1. A complete medical and ophthalmic history is obtained.

Selection Criteria

Patient Selection for Radial Keratotomy

1. Age 18 to 80.

2. Myopia greater than 2.0D.

3. Must be symptomatic (with difficulty with CLs and glasses).

4. Must be well motivated.

5. Must have realistic expectations.

Patient Selection for Astigmatic Keratotomy

1. Astigmatism with-the-rule greater than 2.5D.

2. Astigmatism against-the-rule greater than 2.0D.

3. Must be symptomatic.

4. Must be well motivated.

5. Must have realistic expectations.

Additional Patient Criteria

1. The myopia should be relatively stable. If worn, hard contacts must be left out of the eyes for three to four weeks to allow time for the corneas to become stable. Soft lenses must be left out for one week.

2. Corneas must be normal by slit-lamp exam and by topography. Keratoscopy and keratometry are not enough.

Range for RK and AK

The nomograms in this book have been found to be effective up to about 8 diopters myopia and astigmatism with fairly high predictability. The accuracy and predictability is greatest in mild to moderate myopia, that is, up to about 6 diopters. From 6 to 8 diopters and above, the accuracy becomes more dependent on the surgeon's skill and experience with modifying the nomograms for higher degrees of error.

The patient is advised that the worst eye or the non-dominant eye will be operated on first. If the results are not optimal, the surgical parameters can be adjusted and the redesigned surgery can then be performed on the dominant eye, giving this eye a better chance for a satisfactory result with its first procedure.

Work-up

1. Medical history.
2. Ophthalmic history.
3. Autorefraction.
4. Autokeratometry (Figure 3-2).
5. Topography (Figure 3-3).
6. Patient Education Concepts Informed Consent video and quiz (Figure 3-4).
7. Complete ophthalmologic exam, with cycloplegic refraction (Figure 3-5).
8. Question and answer session with the physician.
9. Pachymetry (Figure 3-6).
10. Arrangement of insurance coverage or financing.
11. Schedule surgery (the calculations and surgical planning are done later).

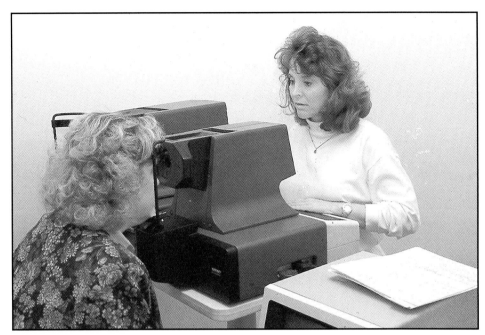

Figure 3-2. Autorefraction and Autokeratometry.

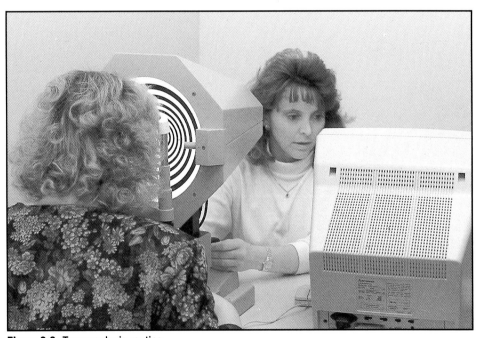

Figure 3-3. Topography is routine.

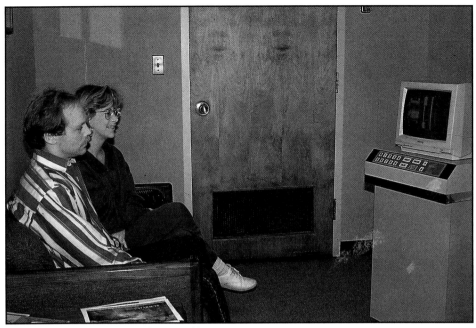

Figure 3-4. Viewing Informed Consent video.

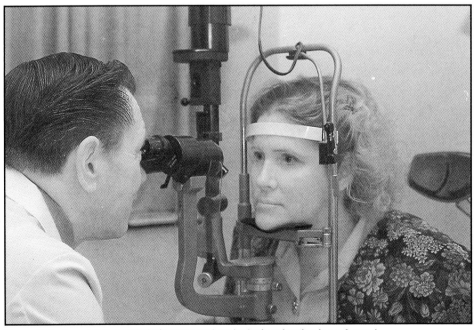

Figure 3-5. A complete ophthalmic exam and cycloplegic refraction is performed.

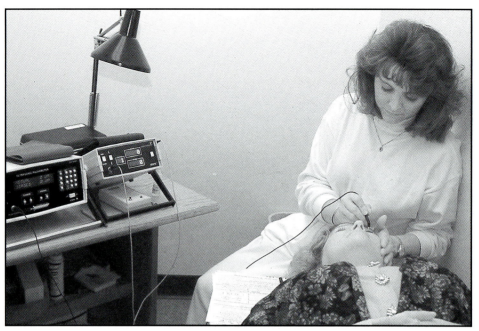

Figure 3-6. Pachymetry is performed in the office prior to surgery.

Patient Information

The object of our sequence of steps in selecting, interviewing, reviewing, and obtaining an informed consent is to be sure that the patient understands and agrees with the following.

1. The relative safety, effectiveness and predictability have been demonstrated in a number of prospective and retrospective studies, but refractive surgery cannot be precisely predicted in any specific case.

2. Glasses or contact lenses may still be required after surgery for best vision.

3. Refractive surgery does not alter the normal aging process of the eye.

4. Reading glasses will be required at some point as the patient gets older.

To explain the process of selection, evaluation, and the surgery itself to patients, families and other concerned individuals or agencies, it is helpful to have typical letters and forms prepared for immediate use. In Appendix C you will find sample letters to patients and insurance companies, patient evaluation and informed consent forms, patient preparation and preoperative instructions, pre and post-op order forms, surgery records and operative reports. Over the years we have found these to be extremely helpful, and they can be easily modified for your own use.

Summary

In the final analysis, the success of radial keratotomy and astigmatic keratotomy depends not on the achievement of 20/20 or 20/40 vision, but on the satisfaction of the patient. Over-promotion of RK as a means of eliminating the patient's need for glasses or contact lenses can only result in a large percentage of dissatisfied patients whose expectations have not and could not have been met.

With proper patient counseling and careful attention to the details of proper surgical planning, most patients will be happy and you will be rewarded with greater success.

4

The Radial Keratotomy Nomogram

A nomogram is a codified table of values based on combinations of physical and theoretical factors which determine the surgical approach for a targeted result. The values derived from these modifiers are based on clinically proven guidelines developed by retrospective study of a large number of cases in the hands of the nomogram designer and those following its systematic approach precisely. For comparable results therefore the surgeon using this nomogram must use the techniques and instrumentation for which the nomogram was designed (Table 4-1).

This method assumes a 90% achieved *average* depth of incisions with the incisions being carried centrifugally (i.e., from the optical zone to the limbus) and is based on the American method of making incisions from the optical zone with an American style diamond blade (sharp on the slanted edge) and optical zone markers measured from the *outside*.

Refractions are based on cycloplegic refraction and the modifying factors considered, in addition to refractive error, are age, keratometry, sex, intraocular pressure, corneal thickness and corneal diameter. The sum of these factors added to or subtracted from the actual refractive error gives the theoretical or working sphere.

Table 4-1.
Thornton Nomogram for Radial Keratotomy

Requisites: Centrifugal incisions, cycloplegic refraction, 90% achieved *average* depth (98% at OZ) and redeepening of all radial incisions for increased effect when indicated (see below).

Factors considered: Refractive Error, Age, Sex, Intraocular Pressure, Corneal Thickness, Corneal Diameter and Keratometry.
The sum of all these factors = the working sphere (theoretical)

Age: For every year below age 30 add 2% to the myopic error. For every year above age 30 subtract 2% from the myopic error to age 50, then 1% per year thereafter to age 75.

Sex: Subtract 3 years from age for premenopausal females to age 40.

IOP: For every mm IOP below 12 add 2% to the myopic refractive error. For every mm IOP above 15, subtract 2% from the myopic refractive error.

Corneal Thickness: For central corneal thickness less than 490 μ, add 10% to the myopia. From 490 to 510, add 5%. From 510 to 580 make no change. From 580 to 600, subtract 5%, and above 600 subtract 10% from the myopia.

Corneal Diameter: If the corneal diameter is less than 11.5 mm, add 10% to the myopic error. If the corneal diameter is greater than 12.5 mm, subtract 10% from the myopic error.

Keratometry: If the average K is 42.75 or less, add 10% to the myopia. From 42.75 to 43.50, add 5%. From 43.50 to 46.00, make no change. From 46.00 to 46.75, subtract 5%. If the average K is 46.75 or more, subtract 10% from the myopia.

Advanced Radial Keratotomy Technique: Titration of Effect

Four incisions would be expected to give results in the lower half of any given range and eight would be expected to give results in the upper half. Back-cutting or "Squaring up" from the limbus will assure the maximum correction possible with a single pass in any given optical zone. *Redeepening* increases the effect from 0.50 to 0.75D with either 4 or 8 incisions. Deepening all incisions to 98% from the 7mm optical zone adds approximately 0.50D to the correction and deepening to 98% from the 5mm optical zone adds approximately 0.75D to the correction.

Table 4-1. (continued)
Thornton Nomogram for Radial Keratotomy

Theoretical Working Sphere Range of Myopic Power	Optical Zone (Number of Incisions in parentheses)
0.75 — 1.12	5.00 (8) 4.75 (4)
1.13 — 1.49	4.75 (8) 4.50 (4)
1.50 — 2.11	4.50 (8) 4.25 (4)
2.12 — 2.61	4.25 (8) 4.00 (4)
2.62 — 3.11	4.00 (8) 3.75 (4)
3.12 — 3.73	3.75 (8) 3.50 (4)
3.75 — 4.36	3.50 (8) 3.25 (4)
4.37 — 5.11	3.25 (8) 3.00 (4)
5.12 — 6.11	3.00 (8)
6.12 — 7.50	3.00 (8 & redeepen to 98% from 5mm OZ)
7.51 — 8.00 or more	3.00 (8 & redeepen to 98% from 5 and 7mm OZ)

Table 4-2.
Radial Keratotomy Evaluation Form

Spencer P. Thornton, MD, FACS

Name _____   DOB _____   Date _____

VA s Rx: OD 20/   OS 20/   VA c Rx: OD 20/   OS 20/   Dominant Eye _____

Last Rx: Date _____   OD _____−_____ ×   OS _____−_____ ×

Current Refraction in − Cyl form   OD _____−_____ ×   OS _____−_____ ×

Spherical Equivalent   OD _____   OS _____

Keratometry (Automatic)   OD ___×___ / ___×___   OS ___×___ / ___×___

Keratometry (Manual)   OD ___×___ / ___×___   OS ___×___ / ___×___

IOP: OD ____   OS ____   Diameter: OD ____   OS ____   Axial Length: OD____   OS____

| OD | PACHYMETRY | OS |

3mm Avg _____		3mm Avg _____
5mm Avg _____		5mm Avg _____
7mm Avg _____		7mm Avg _____

Age ____ Sex ____ = ± %_____   OD Working Sphere _____ OS Working Sphere _____

IOP, Pach, Diam, AvgK = ± %_____   OD Working Cylinder _____ OS Working Cylinder _____

Total Sph Modifier % = ± %_____

Cyl Modifier % ($^{1}/_{4}$ Sph) = ± %_____

OD: OZ _____ mm No._____   OS: OZ _____ mm No._____

Blade setting _____ µ   Blade setting _____ µ

Redeepen @ 5 to _____ µ @ 7 to_____ µ   Redeepen @ 5 to _____ µ @ 7 to_____ µ

___ "T" Incisions_____ °Axis ___ °Depth ___ µ   ___ "T" Incisions_____ °Axis ___ °Depth ___ µ

Modifiers: Sex, IOP, Corneal Thickness (Pach), Diameter, Keratometry (Average K): See Nomogram

Why Doesn't One Size Fit All?

For the first few years after intraocular lenses were introduced in the United States, many "experts" were advising using only one power of intraocular lens for everyone. "Nineteen diopters will take care of more than ninety percent of the patients," we were told. It didn't take long for us to realize that it was just not that simple. There were a number of factors which influenced the visual outcome with lens implants, and over a period of years the formulas were modified and refined to bring about more accurate results.

Just as we have learned to individualize intraocular lens implants for our cataract patients based on a number of variables, so too have we learned that there are a number of factors which influence the outcome of refractive surgery.

The Role of Modifiers

Why use modifiers at all? Why not just use two or three optical zones and one set length of the blade and vary the size of the optical zone only by the amount of myopia present, with, say, a large optical zone for errors up to 2 diopters, a second, medium sized optical zone for errors from 2 to 4 diopters, and a small optical zone for errors of over 4 diopters? Then, use four incisions for all cases with the plan that if more effect was needed, you could add four more incisions at the original optical zone.

The fact is, a fair number of cases could do fairly well with this plan. And indeed, some surgeons have done just as described above and claim "good results."

If you limit your practice primarily to one demographic group and a relatively small range of powers you could get by with a simplistic nomogram like this too, but the real world is not limited to one age group and a small range of myopic powers. It is diverse, and consists of all ages, a great range of powers, and other variables such as gender, genetic differences in corneal structure, varying astigmatism, different intraocular pressures, etc.

Custom Tailored Surgery

Using modifiers in surgical planning allows personalization and greater precision in surgery. Surgery for myopia and astigmatism should be tailored to the patient, not the patient to the surgery. By discovering and utilizing the differences in tissue characteristics from eye to eye one has the opportunity of individualizing the procedure. But this takes thought and planning. It is not a cook-book approach.

The prime concern for the surgeon beginning the study of radial and astigmatic keratotomy is that he or she be given a nomogram for surgical planning which is reasonable, straightforward and easily understood, so that he or she can get an overall feeling of how the operation works without being limited to a simplistic mathematical grid which gives an inaccurate projection as to the accuracy of the operation.

Over-simplification and trivialization of RK and AK have caused a number of good surgeons to become disillusioned with the procedures, not because they are not valid procedures, but because they put their faith in a system that is flawed and instruments and devices that were sold as part of the system "without which they could not succeed."

Why Would a Nomogram be Modified?

Nomograms are modified from time to time for several reasons.

1. When continuing data analysis shows a consistent variation from the projected value or result. For example, corneal thickness in the lower and upper range (below 510μ and above 580μ) has been shown to be a consistent modifier, decreasing the effect in shallower corneas and increasing the effect in thicker corneas.

2. When a modifier, on review, acts differently from that previously understood, as in astigmatism and the cornea's response to transverse incisions (the direct and more immediate relaxing effect of transverse incisions as opposed to the secondary stretching with radial incisions).

3. When a new method or approach alters the projections, as with arcuate incisions compared to straight transverse incisions with increased effect and greater coupling with arcuate incisions of the same chord length as straight.

4. When refinements in technique and instrumentation allow greater precision in the procedure. An example of this is the greater precision allowed with 360° arcuate markers for transverse incisions as compared to other press-on "cut-on-the-line" markers, and measuring lengths in degrees of arc rather than in millimeters.

5. When a modifier, on review of a great number of cases, is seen to have a consistent bearing on the outcome—such as corneal diameter and the resulting difference in relative length of the radial incisions.

6. When a new modifier is discovered and analyzed, and found to have significant bearing on the surgical plan. An example of this is corneal topography and corneal mapping with the discovery of astigmatic asymmetry which requires modification of the nomograms to allow for asymmetric surgical approaches.

The Surgical Plan

Surgery for myopia and astigmatism should be adapted to the patient, rather than adapting the patient to the surgery. The nomogram and its modifiers should be carefully followed. To ignore known modifiers is to assure imprecision and the necessity of repeat "enhancement" surgery.

I have been involved in an ongoing study to determine the relative importance of the various modifiers in influencing the accuracy of the surgical plan for radial keratotomy and, to no one's surprise, found that when each variable was analyzed with all others held constant, myopia alone accounted for 60% or more of the relative value of everything influencing the surgical planning of radial keratotomy. If you then added variable age you accounted for around 80% of the factors influencing the accuracy of RK surgery.

What this means is that if you used only the amount of myopia and the patient's age to determine the size of the optical zone, and used a standard, unvarying blade depth and ignored corneal thickness, gender, keratometry, corneal diameter, intraocular pressure and any other variables, you could be within one diopter of emmetropia in about four out of five cases. Put another way, all of the other modifiers account for about 20% of the accuracy of refractive surgery.

When intraocular pressure, gender, corneal thickness, keratometry and corneal diameter are added to age and myopia, the number of cases brought to within one diopter of emmetropia on the first procedure increases. For example, intraocular pressure was normal or "average" in the majority of cases, but in 7% the intraocular pressure was an outlier (high or low) and in those cases the intraocular pressure affected the amount of surgery to be performed. Multiple factors were considered separately and because of this the total modifier effect adds up to more than 100%.

The following shows the relative effect of the modifiers in the Thornton system.

Myopia = 60%
Age = 22%
Gender (Sex) = 15%
Intraocular Pressure = 7%
Keratometry = 6%
Corneal Thickness = 6%
Corneal Diameter = 4%
Unknown Biological Variables = 5%

Theoretically at least, using all of the known modifiers would appear to bring one closer to the targeted correction in a significantly higher percentage of cases.

If verified in other studies, these findings may account for the differences in response from one system nomogram to another in which fewer modifiers are used. It may also determine the variation in effect that keeps one eye from responding to a given amount of surgery in the way another one does in the same individual.

What Are the Modifiers and How Do They Affect Outcomes?

Other than the refractive error itself, **age** is the most important modifier. Since nomograms are based on a thirty year old, for every year below age 30 add 2% to the myopic error. For every year above age 30 subtract 2% from the myopic error to age 50, then 1% per year thereafter to age 75. The loss of elastic recovery of aging tissues appears to level off after age 75.

Sex or gender can have an effect on surgical outcomes because of hormonal differences. Premenopausal women react as if they are about three years younger than their actual age. Therefore age should be reduced by about three years for women up to age 40.

The effect of relaxing incisions is enhanced by any factor that increases the stretching of the cornea. The **intraocular pressure** is one of these factors and the greater the **IOP** the greater the corneal "stretch." The nomogram assumes a "normal" IOP range of 12 to 15mm, therefore, for every millimeter of IOP below 12, add 2% to the myopic refractive error. For every millimeter of IOP above 15, subtract 2% from the myopic refractive error.

As one would expect, thinner corneas do not react to the same degree as thicker corneas with deep corneal incisions. Therefore, if the central **corneal thickness** is less than 490μ, add 10% to the myopia. From 490μ to 510μ, add 5%. From 510μ to 580μ make no change. From 580μ to 600μ, subtract 5%, and above 600μ subtract 10% from the myopic error.

Within certain limits, the **corneal diameter**, or length of the incision, determines the effect. Larger corneas allow relatively longer incisions from any given optical zone to the limbus, allowing more "spread" of the incision and greater "stretch" of the central cornea. Conversely, smaller corneas limit the incision lengths from the optical zone to the limbus. To compensate for these differences, if the corneal diameter is less than 11.5mm, add 10% to the myopic error. If the corneal diameter is greater than 12.5mm, subtract 10% from the myopic error. If you do not carry your radial incisions to the limbus, this modifier is meaningless.

Regarding **keratometry**, the flatter K reading represents the spherical component of the myopia and the steeper K represents the cylinder. The average K represents the "spherical equivalent." The nomogram assumes an average corneal curvature of from 43.50 to 46.00 diopters. To compensate for steeper or flatter corneas the nomogram is modified as follows: If the average K is 42.75 or less, add

10% to the myopia. From 42.75 to 43.50, add 5%. From 43.50 to 46.00 make no change. From 46.00 to 46.75, subtract 5%, and if the average K is 46.75 or more, subtract 10% from the myopia.

Using the Modifiers

The sum of all of the factors (modifiers) given above, is added to or subtracted from the actual myopic error, giving a theoretical or "working" sphere on which the nomogram is based. The result is known as the "theoretical error."

Even though a modifier may lie in the "normal" range and not need to be used in individual calculations, it has been allowed for in the nomogram. The difference between modifier power and overall modifier effect should not be confused. The "effect" is a function of its application, and the normal effect is calculated into the nomogram.

For ease of calculation the nomogram is designed to apply a modifier only when its value is out of the "normal" range. If a value is not entered for any given modifier, it is assumed to be "average" or "normal" and defaults to the normal average value in the nomogram. It should be obvious to the reader that even within the "normal range" a variable effect is possible.

The Nomogram Applied

Practically speaking, no nomogram is accurate to a quarter diopter or even a half diopter. There are too many *surgeon* variables. But as you gain experience—and confidence—your results will become more reproducible.

The basic Thornton RK Nomogram gives a range of power with each optical zone and the higher the error the wider the range. This leaves some latitude within each range for variable response to the surgery.

It is possible for the surgeon, with careful planning and attention to technique, to further determine the amount of response. This response can be titrated in several ways: by "squaring up" the ends of each incision, by deepening the incisions at any of several optical zones or by varying the number of incisions.

Titration for Increased Precision

"Squaring Up" and Secondary Optical Zones

Four incisions would be expected to give results in the lower half of any given range, and eight would be expected to give results in the upper half. Back-cutting or "squaring up" the incisions in the periphery (at the limbus) assures that the amount corrected will be in the mid portion of the range targeted in the nomogram

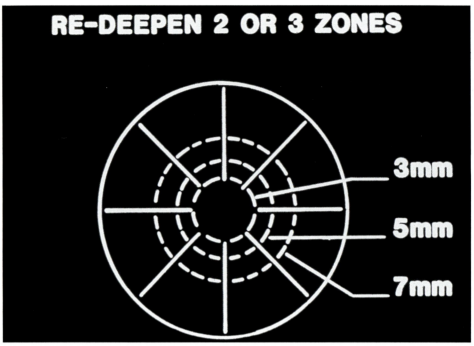

Figure 4-1. Secondary optical zones allow titration of effect.

for any given optical zone. If a greater amount of correction is desired, one can increase the effect of the incisions using the same optical zone by deepening the incisions from any *secondary* optical zone, the amount of increased effect determined by the size of the secondary optical zone.

Redeepening for Increased Effect

By utilizing the 5 and the 7mm secondary optical zones, the surgeon can *titrate* and increase incrementally the effect of incisions from any given primary optical zone. Redeepening all incisions to 98% depth from the 7mm optical zone with a 4 radial pattern will give an increase in effect of approximately 0.50D, or about 5%, and approximately 0.75D with an 8 radial pattern (Figure 4-1).

Redeepening a 4 radial pattern to 98% depth from the 5mm optical zone will give an increased effect of approximately 0.75D, or about 10%. Redeepening eight radials to 98% from both the 5 and the 7mm OZ will give an increased effect of from 1 to 1.25D, or about 15% additional effect.

Since deepening (redeepening) produces a "shelf" at the base of the incision from the point redeepened, and this shelf may diffract light and produce glare, it is advised to keep the secondary optical zone outside the range of the normally dilated pupil and the 5mm optical zone is usually the smallest secondary optical zone recommended (Figures 4-2, 4-3, and 4-4).

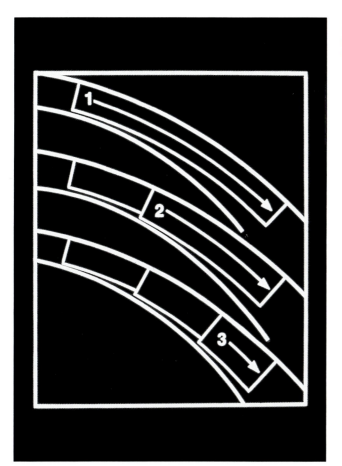

Figure 4-2. Deepening produces a shelf at the base of the incision.

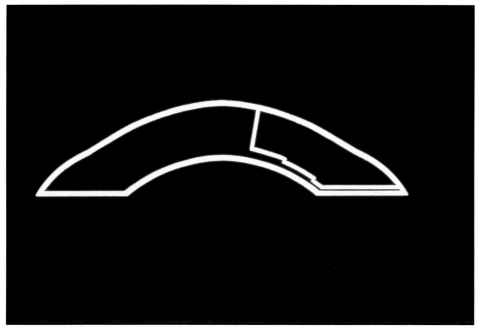

Figure 4-3. 5mm should be the smallest redeepening zone because of "steps."

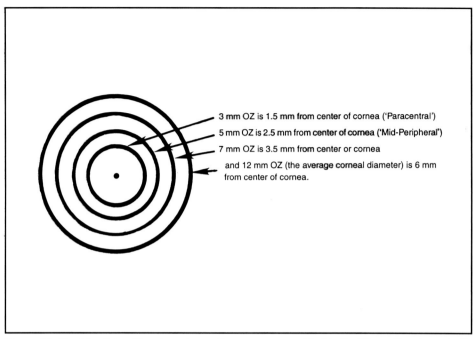

Figure 4-4. Most "peripheral" pachymetry readings are measured inside the 12mm diameter, actually closer to the 11mm diameter (the 11mm OZ), 5.5mm from the center of the cornea. If a radial incision begins at the 3mm OZ (1.5mm from the center of the cornea) and is carried to the "periphery" (the 11mm OZ) its maximum length will be 4mm.

Summary

To achieve the best results with this nomogram you must use the specific surgical techniques and system of instruments for which the nomogram was designed. With care and careful adherence to proper surgical planning, the results of your refractive surgery can be more accurately determined and bring a great deal of pleasure to you and your patients.

5

Instruments for Refractive Surgery

Accurate RK and AK surgery depend on quality instrumentation as well as skillful surgery. The surgeon has the right and the responsibility to demand the best in instrumentation from the instrument and device maker. He should not be taken in by the sales pitch of any company representative selling "a complete system" of instruments and devices which will guarantee his success. He should carefully study the available instruments and devices, check with other physician users whose advice he trusts, and get a satisfaction guarantee from any dealer selling equipment.

The instruments that I discuss in this chapter are those that I have personally used and have found effective for the task for which they were designed. I have no direct or indirect financial interest in any instrument or any instrument manufacturer, and I do not receive payment for recommending any instrument, even those that bear my name.

The refractive surgeon, whether beginner or advanced, should purchase the very best in instrumentation. The ease and accuracy with which you perform delicate and precise corneal incisions are dependent on the accuracy and reliability of your instruments. Don't skimp here!

The most important instrument in refractive surgery is the diamond blade. All other instruments are designed to define it's accuracy, proper placement, precision with which it passes through tissue, and the pattern of incisions it makes.

Optical zone markers define the blade's position and placement. The micro meter handle and footplates determine the accuracy of its depth in tissue. Fixation instruments determine the precision with which it passes through the cornea, and radial and astigmatic markers determine the pattern of incisions.

All instruments are not the same. Quality differences between manufacturers is the rule rather than the exception. It is also important to remember that a certificate of accuracy means nothing after an instrument has been used. It must be properly cared for. In the following pages I will describe the instruments I use and recommend.

Instruments

The instrument set for RK and AK should include the following:

> Wire speculum
> Angled 0.12 Forceps
> Thornton Fixation Ring
> Radial Marker - 6 Line
> Radial Marker - 8 Line
> Thornton Optical Zone Markers from 3.0 mm to 5.0 mm in quarter mm
> steps, plus a 6.0, 7.0 and 8.0 mm marker
> Press-on 360° Arcuate Marker
> Thornton Incision Spreader
> Thornton Step Gauge
> American Diamond Micrometer Knife with 35° blade
> Thornton Triple Edged Arcuate Diamond Micrometer Knife
> Instrument Holder
> 27 Gauge Blunt Tip Irrigating Canula

A number of fine instrument companies manufacture these instruments to strict specifications, but be sure that the instruments are certified to conform to the designs as described in the following pages.

Angled 0.12 Microfixation Forceps: These forceps are used for gentle fixation of the globe during marking of the cornea with optical zone or astigmatic corneal markers (I recommend angle-tipped microfixation forceps with 0.12mm teeth).

When one uses microfixation forceps, particularly of the Colebri type, one is aware that he is looking down the sharply angled tip, perpendicular to the teeth, and the actual point of grasping tissue is obscured. With an angle of approximately 23° at the tip, the teeth of these delicate forceps can be seen easily as it grasps tissue even when used in the left hand reaching across the cornea.

6 Line and 8 Line Low Profile Markers: With the Thornton low profile markers approximately 2mm in height, the centration around the previously marked center and optical zone ring can be easily placed binocularly, eliminating the parallax problems with higher markers (Figure 5-1). Markers are available in both stainless steel and titanium.

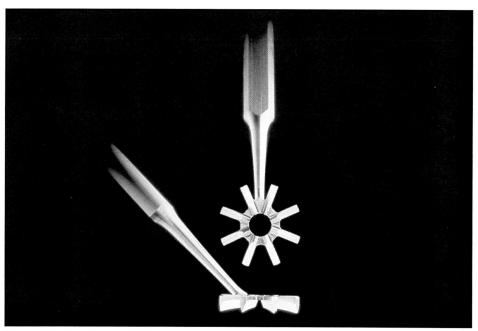

Figure 5-1. 8 line low profile RK marker.

Optical Zone Markers: The optical zone markers I recommend are ultra-thin, measuring only about 1.5mm in height. The measurement of optical zone size is made from the outside diameter, i.e. the markers are beveled from the inside toward the outside so that the outside is flat (Figure 5-2). This is important in obtaining accurate measurements precisely from the optical zone marker, as it is easier to cut precisely from the outside of the optical zone mark than from the inside.

With these ultra-thin markers the parallax problems of higher markers are done away with and marking of the optical zone can be done binocularly rather than monocularly. Optical zone markers are available in 0.25mm increments from 3.0 to 5.0mm and also 6mm, 7mm and 8mm (Figures 5-3 and 5-4).

The Fixation Ring: With one or two point fixation during refractive surgery, the globe tends to move when the blade is passed either from the limbus toward the optical zone, or from the optical zone out toward the limbus. This is especially noticeable after the first and second incisions when more pressure is necessary to assure adequate depth. Even with two point fixation on either side of the cornea, skew and deviation of incisions are quite common (Figures 5-5 and 5-6).

The Thornton Fixation Ring with its 16mm internal diameter provides sure fixation of the globe with atraumatic teeth providing excellent stabilization and allowing adequate pressure on the globe as each incision is being made to assure full depth. Eight markings on the ring serve as a guide for directing the cuts.

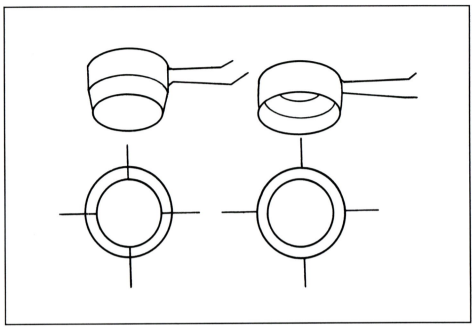

Figure 5-2. Incisions are more precisely made when starting at the outside of the OZ mark.

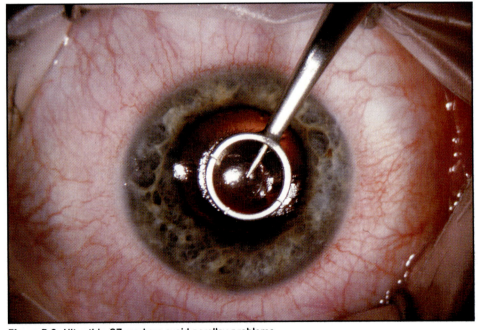

Figure 5-3. Ultra thin OZ markers avoid parallax problems.

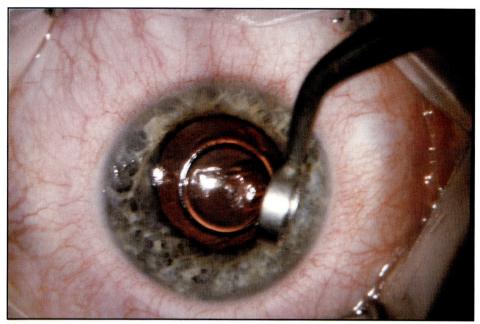

Figure 5-4. Thornton OZ markers are measured on outside diameter.

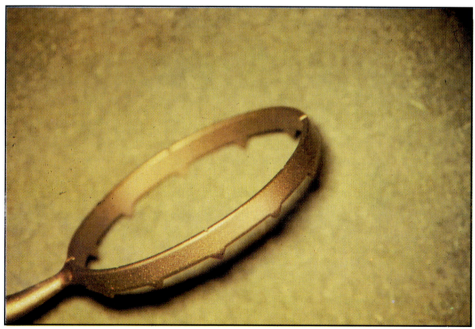

Figure 5-5. Thornton Fixation Ring.

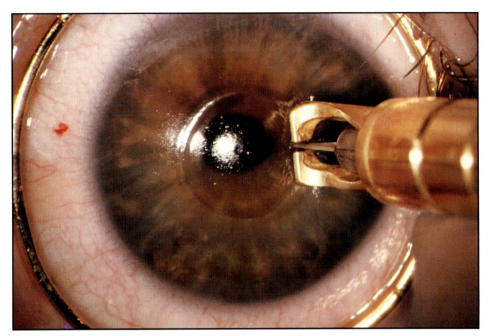

Figure 5-6. The fixation ring stabilizes eye as incisions are made.

Incision Spreading Forceps: Examining the depth and length of corneal incisions to visually confirm adequate incision characteristics must be done gently and without overspreading the incision. The Thornton incision spreading forceps are designed to safely spread and examine the corneal incision, a stop incorporated in the handle prevents the forceps tips from spreading more than 1mm, and sandblasted tips afford safe, yet sure retraction.

The sandblasted outside of the blades of the tips have another use. In preparation for suturing overcorrections, when incisions must be opened to remove cellular ingrowth, the sandblasted edges of the spreading forceps provide a gently debriding surface to scrape the incision walls (Figure 5-7).

The Diamond Blade: The best blade for radial incisions is the 30° American style diamond blade with a dull vertical back edge, because of it's safety in inserting it at the optical zone. For all other incisions— transverse, arcuate, and back cutting for reduction of radial optical zone size—the Triple Edged Arcuate (Thornton TEA) diamond blade is best. All three edges are sharp—the vertical edge, the 200 squared bottom edge, and the 15° angled edge. This blade was designed to be able to turn in tissue with minimal effort, and its 200 flat bottom edge acts as a rudder which helps it to "track" well in tissue (Figure 5-8).

The triple-edged diamond knives which are now available feature footplates that are long enough to applanate the cornea on either side of the blade, yet thin enough to allow visualization of the blade through the microscope.

With the thin triple-edged diamond, the blade passes into corneal tissue with almost no resistance, and by moving the blade in either direction, any length

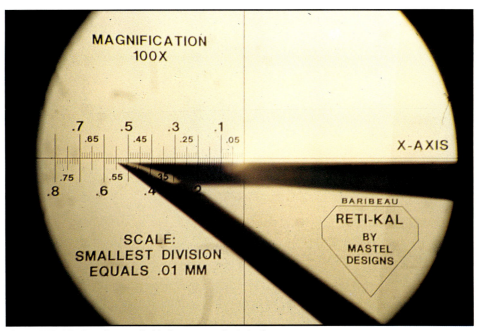

Figure 5-7. 30° American style blade cuts on slanted edge.

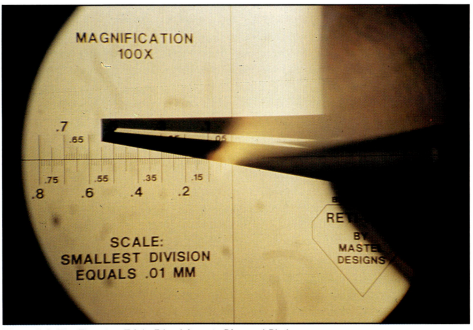

Figure 5-8. The Thornton Triple-Edged Arcuate Diamond Blade.

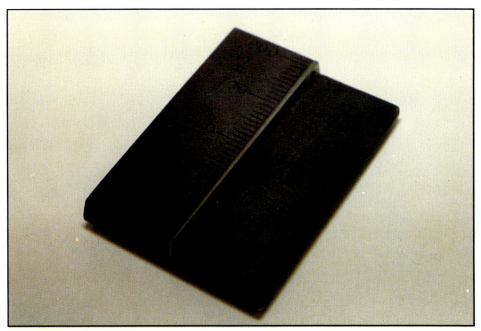

Figure 5-9. The Step Gauge.

incision can be produced with accuracy and assurance that full depth is achieved at each end of the incision.

With secure ring fixation the triple-edged diamond blade has been found useful for all incisions, including the American style radial incisions carried from the optical zone to the limbus. One caution: because its bottom edge is extremely sharp, it tends to cut deeply without additional pressure. Movements must therefore be made very slowly so that when microperforations occur they can't become *macro*perforations.

The triple-edged arcuate diamond blade is available in the United States from Doug Mastel at Mastel Designs and from Storz Instrument Co., and in Europe from Anton Meyer at Meyco.

The Step Gauge: Intraoperative measurement of blade extension is aided by the use of a step gauge. This is a small measuring block with a shelving "step" along the side against which the fingers holding the micrometer knife handle can rest. A bar-scale, accurate to within 5μ, with marks every 10μ (1/100th mm) allows rapid confirmation of the extension of the blade in the micrometer handle (Figures 5-9 and 5-10).

The Instrument Holder: The most frequent cause of damage to diamond blades is contact with metal handles of other instruments on the surgical instrument tray. No matter how carefully the surgeon places his diamond blade on the tray, there is always the possibility that it will accidentally make contact with other instruments on the tray during surgery.

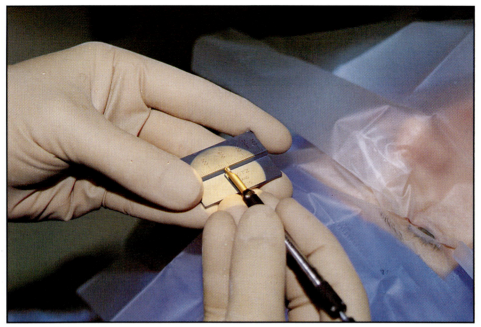

Figure 5-10. Measuring blade extension on the step gauge during surgery.

An instrument holder has been designed to avoid the possibility of damage by keeping diamond knives separate and secure on the instrument table. The device is an anodyzed aluminum block with two pairs of V-shaped depressions designed to hold micrometer blade handles securely above the level of the instrument table so no contact with other instruments is possible. The block is designed to allow easy access to the instruments and take up minimal space on the instrument tray (Figure 5-11). The Double V instrument holder is available in the United States from Mastel Designs.

Other Equipment: In addition to these instruments there is another device that is of utmost importance in determining the accuracy and quality of the diamond blade, and that is the calibration and inspection microscope.

All microscopes are not the same. I've used several brands of microscopes for inspection and calibration of my diamond blades for surgery and have been fairly pleased with them. But there have been drawbacks. In studying the features of each, I've developed a set of recommendations for the surgeon looking for a dependable RK microscope.

The RK Microscope: In looking for a calibration and inspection microscope you should demand one with a removable knife holder that locks the knife in place for sterilization. Its also good to get one that protects the knife if the holder is accidentally dropped. When the knife is placed on the microscope stage the holder should positively lock in place so that there is precise alignment and no movement.

The working distance, from the bottom of the objective lens to the blade, should

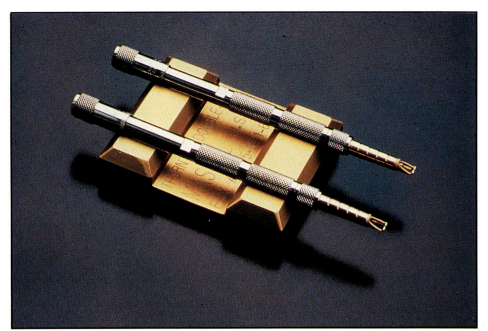

Figure 5-11. The Thornton "Double V" instrument holder.

be no less than 30mm to avoid possible contact with the knife.

The illumination system should allow fully lighted inspection from all angles, not just a silhouette. A dual halogen illumination system with variable intensity is preferred, even if a separate side light is necessary.

The depth of field will vary with power and I want to be able to find the blade quickly, so I like a variable power, preferably with a zoom lens. It's desirable for the highest power to be in the 80x to 100x range, but, for all but the most critical high power examinations, the most useful calibration power is in the 30x to 50x range, and for inspection the most useful power is in the 80x to 90x range. A single power microscope does not offer the versatility needed for accurate intra-operative blade examination.

For greater precision, an electronic micrometer, accurate to one micron resolution, is preferred to a reticle. It is much easier to use and doesn't require interpretation (Figure 5-12).

I recently discovered an RK microscope that meets all of the criteria I've looked for in accuracy and ease of use for diamond blade calibration and inspection. It's the Marinoff calibration-inspection microscope. This microscope is a delight to use with its precision zoom optics and adjustable eyepiece. It offers halogen dual illumination within the microscope body, and its greater depth of field, the best I've seen, makes accurate calibration a breeze. The Marinoff RK Microscope is available in the United States from G & G Medical Instruments Ltd, P.O. Box 547, Fort Montgomery, NY, 10922.

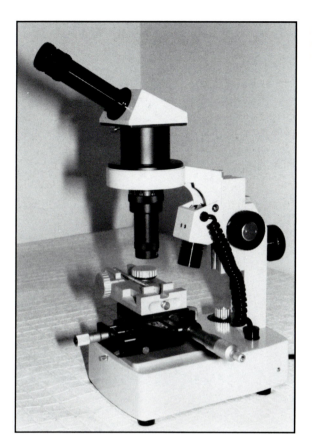

Figure 5-12. The Marinoff Calibration, Inspection Microscope.

Cleaning Diamond Knives

Immediately after use in surgery, and before the diamond has time to dry, rinse the blade with sterile water. Blood or cellular debris can be rinsed off by using a squirt bottle. It is important to point the tip of the knife toward the floor to allow gravity to drain the fluid away from the internal shaft of the handle where contaminants can accumulate.

If vigorous rinsing fails to remove debris adequately, the surgeon can gently push the blade into a wet cellulose sponge, wiping the sides of the diamond. Be careful to avoid lateral pressure on the stone as it can fracture. Move the diamond in the direction it was designed to move. Stabbing the extended blade into a styrofoam peanut which has been wet with detergent soap may be effective in removing proteinaceous buildup. It must then be copiously rinsed with deionized distilled water and then inspected under the inspection-calibration microscope. It is important to remove all residual soap or other chemicals used in cleaning to avoid introducing these chemicals in the eye at next use.

6

American vs. Russian Technique

Valid side-by-side comparisons of the American versus the Russian technique are dependent on the researcher's ability to use each method properly. When done correctly, with proper extension of the American blade and ring fixation of the eye, I believe the American system is more precise and reproducible (Figure 6-1).

Advocates of the Russian technique (centripetal incisions using a vertical cutting blade carried from the limbus to the optical zone) claim that this technique produces deeper cuts because of the cutting forces of a vertical edge passing through tissue. By *pushing* the vertical blade through tissue they do not have the degree of control which is an important part of the American technique.

Tissue resistance is greater on the perpendicular knife edge and the surgeon unconsciously pushes the blade more firmly into tissue. Tissue resistance is less on a slanted knife edge and pressure must be deliberately maintained. With firm, slow pressure, the slanted edge blade cuts as deep or deeper and with greater control and greater safety.

With the Russian technique (going from the limbus to the optical zone) using both hands to guide the knife without the use of a fixation ring for stability, control of fine movements of the eye is sacrificed and the chance of crossing the boundary of the clear optical zone is present with every incision. As the optical zone line is approached by the footplates of the blade holder, the optical zone boundary is obscured, making an accurate end-point difficult.

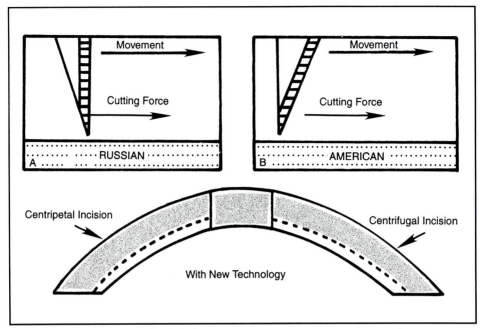

Figure 6-1. American vs. Russian Technique.

With the American technique (cutting with the slanted edge of the blade from the optical zone out to the limbus in one pass of the blade) a more accurate view of the optical zone mark is possible and the tip of the blade can be accurately placed on the optical zone mark at the beginning of every incision. Then, with proper extension of the blade, the incisions can be fully as deep as with a vertical edged blade.

To achieve the same sharp vertical configuration of the incision at the optical zone with the American blade as is claimed with the Russian, the blade is set about 10% longer than pachymetry and "under-cutting" at the optical zone is necessary (Figure 6-2).

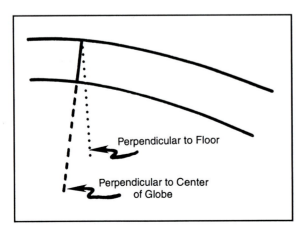

Figure 6-2. Undercutting at the optical zone.

The dull back of the American blade prevents inadvertant entry into the visual axis with resulting greater safety and greater precision (Figure 6-3).

Double-track incisions are inherently less precise than a single pass of the blade. In order to achieve a 90% average depth, an American style blade (sharp on the slanted edge) requires a bias of about 10% (i.e., set about 10% longer than 100% of pachymetry). In order to achieve a 90% incision depth with a Russian style blade (sharp on the vertical edge) pushed toward the optical zone, a 0% bias is used (i.e., the blade is set at 100% of pachymetry).

A recent concession of the "Russian cutters" is the double cutting technique which uses a blade sharp on the slanted side and a short sharp portion on the vertical edge. This blade is inserted at the optical zone, as in the American technique, carried toward the limbus, then reversed and carried back to the optical zone. The claim is that with this back-and-forth cutting they get the safety of the American technique and the deep cuts of the Russian technique.

Cutting one way and then reversing directions introduces an unpredictable and imprecise factor that is dependent on the amount of pressure used to determine depth of the second cut. Therefore, it is impossible to be consistent in depth by using a double cutting blade back and forth in tissue.

Double-track cutting is advocated as a benefit to those surgeons who are using only a single para-central pachymetry reading because they don't achieve optimal incision depth in one or more quadrants to begin with and they are

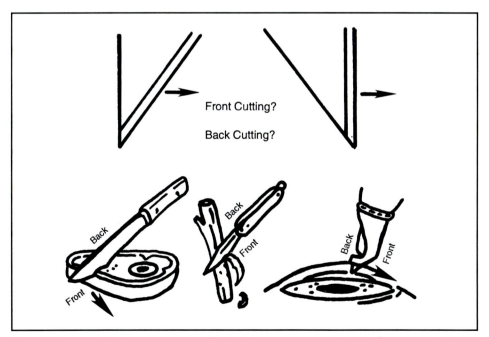

Figure 6-3. By tradition, the front of a knife is the curved part of the blade. Thus the term "front cutting" refers to cutting with the angled edge of the crystal blade, and "back cutting" refers to cutting with the vertical edge.

simply trying to create deeper incisions by cutting back and forth. But don't confuse "deeper" with "more precise." If the incision depth is correct on the first pass, there is no need to double track.

Other Differences

There are other system differences between the American and the Russian techniques which make the American system more precise.

In the Russian system, only *one* "temporal, para-central" pachymetry measurement is taken. In the American system, multiple readings are made in every quadrant so that the depth is known in every part of the cornea where incisions are to be made.

The Russian technique advocates using "the thinnest" corneal measurement, though they do not actually know that the one measurement taken is really in the thinnest area of the cornea.

The Russian system uses only two modifiers, myopia and age. The American system uses all known modifiers for greater precision: myopia, age, IOP, pachymetry, corneal diameter, keratometry and gender.

Because of these differences the American system has been found to be more precise and predictable. Though the American system takes more thought and requires individualization for each patient, the results, with fewer "enhancements" and a wider range of errors correctable, make the extra effort worthwhile.

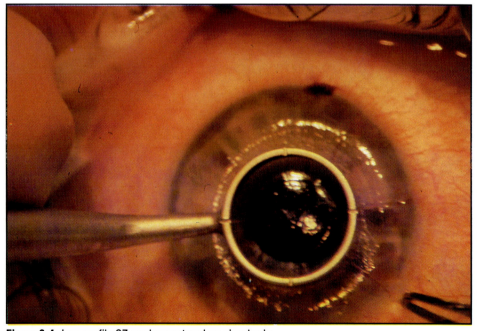

Figure 6-4. Low profile OZ marker centered on visual axis.

The American RK Procedure

1. The eye is anesthesized as described in Chapter 8, *Ocular Anesthesia*.

2. The center of the visual axis is marked under the operating microscope as described in Chapter 9, *Determining the Visual Axis*.

3. The proper optical zone is outlined on the cornea with the low profile marker described in Chapter 5, *Instruments for Refractive Surgery* (Figure 6-4).

4. The Thornton fixation ring is placed on the eye, with light pressure applied as each incision is made, releasing pressure after each incision.

5. The diamond blade, pre-set to the proper depth, is inserted at the edge of the optical zone mark (Figure 6-5) and carried slowly *to*, but not into, the limbus (Figure 6-6) with each incision as described in this chapter.

6. Each subsequent incision is performed as the first with pressure on the fixation ring as the incision is made. Incisions are squared up or redeepened as directed by the nomogram.

7. At the conclusion of incision performance, incisions are inspected for length and depth (Figure 6-7) and irrigated if necessary (Figure 6-8) to remove blood or cellular debris.

8. Another drop of anesthetic, Xylocaine or Marcaine, is instilled and antibiotic drops are instilled.

9. A light pressure dressing is applied to provide comfort and protection overnight.

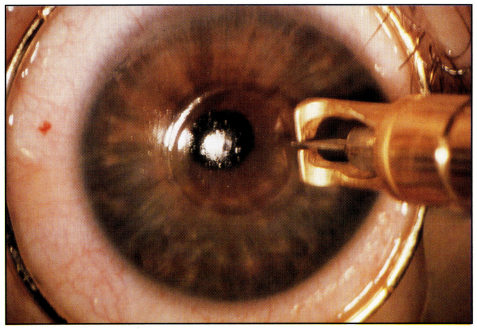

Figure 6-5. American style diamond blade is inserted at OZ and carried slowly toward limbus. Light pressure is applied to fixation ring.

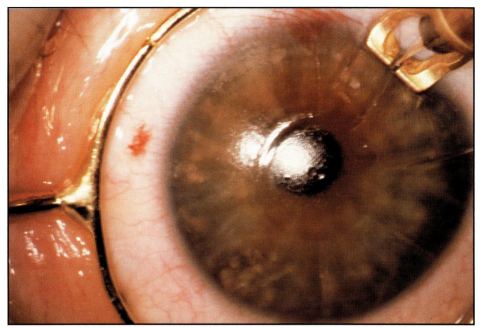

Figure 6-6. Diamond blade is carried *to* but not into the limbus.

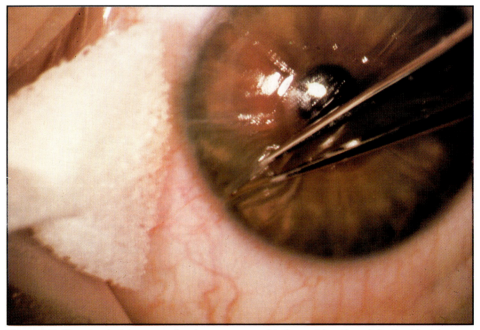

Figure 6-7. Thornton incision spreading forceps are used to inspect length and depth of incisions.

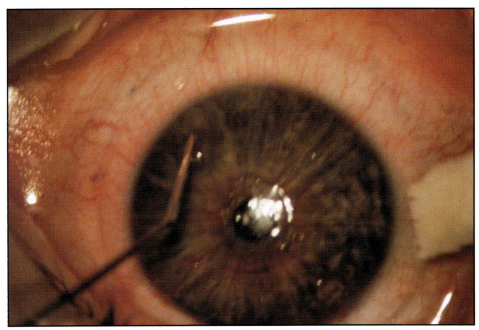

Figure 6-8. Blood and cellular debris may be irrigated from incisions with BSS and 27G bent blunt-tipped canula.

7

Blade Depth and
Number of Incisions

Incision Depth

Depth of incisions *is not* and *should not* be a variable. This nomogram assumes an incision depth of 98% at the optical zone, that is through most of the stroma, almost to Decemet's Membrane, and an average *achieved* incision depth of 85 - 90%. Because of the increasing thickness of the cornea toward the periphery, the percentage depth becomes progressively less over the course of the incision. If the incision begins at 98% depth at the 3mm optical zone and is carried to the limbus, a distance of about 4mm, the average depth will be about 85 - 90% deep.

Determining Maximum Proper Depth

Since the maximum *achieved* depth desired is 90% (that is up to 90% over the length of the radial incision) you must begin with the deepest possible incision depth short of perforation because the percentage will decrease rapidly as you move away from the optical zone (Figure 7-1).

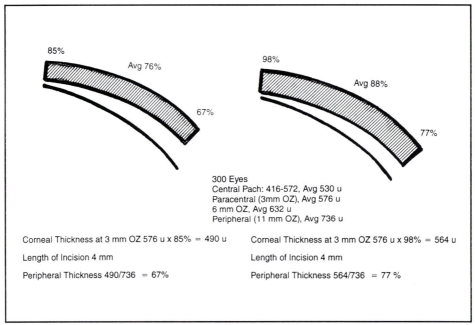

Figure 7-1. Deeper incisions at the optical zone give greater *average* depth.

Setting the Blade Depth

The depth of cut is determined by blade extension. Different diamond blades have different characteristics depending on the blade angle, edge angle, blade width, thickness and blade design (back-cutting, front-cutting, triple-edge, etc.). Therefore I recommend that you start out by setting the blade at 100% of your pachymetry reading at the point of the beginning of the incision. Remember that 98% depth will carry you almost through stroma to Descemet's Membrane and 100% depth will perforate.

Setting the Knife

At the beginning of a day of surgery I calibrate each diamond micrometer knife under the Marinoff calibration-inspection microscope at settings of 0, 500, and 750 microns. Any adjustments in calibration are made at that time (Figure 7-2).

During surgery (after the blade accuracy has been calibrated) I set the diamond blade extension on the micrometer handle and check it after each setting with the step gauge (Figure 7-3).

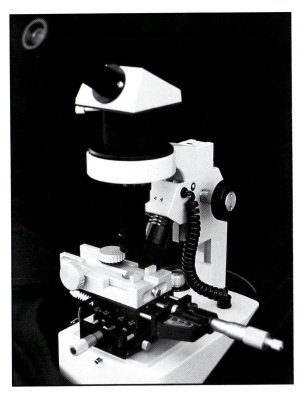

Figure 7-2. The Marinoff RK microscope for pre-operative calibration and inspection.

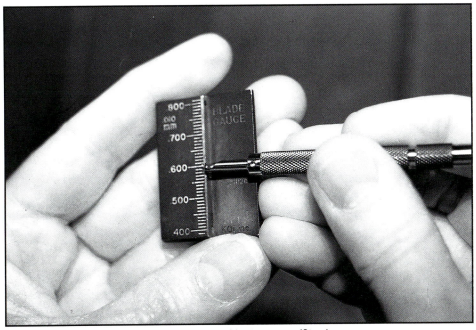

Figure 7-3. Setting the blade depth at surgery with step gauge (Storz).

Your Personal Knife Factor

Use this 100% depth setting on your first several cases. Make your incisions slowly so that if you get a perforation you can stop immediately and it will be a *micro*perforation and not a *macro*perforation. If no perforations occur in the first several cases, or if the incisions appear shallow by slit lamp examination and you are getting undercorrections, extend the blade another 20μ past "100%" and use this "personal knife factor" on your next several cases.

Study your results over the next few cases by slit lamp and refraction. If good results are obtained and the slit lamp confirms your depth, leave this 20μ extension as your personal knife factor for your subsequent cases with this knife. But, if you are still getting undercorrections and have had no microperforations, and you see that the incisions still appear shallow by slit lamp exam, extend the blade another 20μ for your next several cases. Continue to do this until you are satisfied that your knife setting and your pachymetry and "actual corneal depth" are in agreement.

This method of determining your "personal knife factor" should seem familiar to you since all IOL surgeons have done essentially the same thing to determine their "personal A constant" for the particular intraocular lens they are using, calculating and recalculating the variables until their IOL power is predictable.

Number of Incisions

The effect of radial incisions is dependent on their number and length. There is a trade-off between the number of incisions and the optical zone size. It is desirable in younger people with more active pupils to plan for a larger optical zone and so, except for lower myopic errors, an 8-incision pattern will provide this along with greater assurance of full correction of the myopic error. In older patients with less active pupils, a smaller optical zone with four incisions is usually preferred. Four incision patterns usually give results in the lower half of the range and eight incisions give results in the upper part of the range.

Four and eight radial RKs can be supplemented by three and six incision RKs where the four and eight radials correct the upper or lower limits of a refractive range. Three incisions have been found to correct about 80% of the amount of four radials and six radial incisions correct about 80% of that corrected by eight radials. The advantage of using three as opposed to four, and six as opposed to eight radials is the ability to titrate the amount of correction achieved with less fluctuation and glare and greater ease of performance.

Earlier refractive stability seems to be another benefit with fewer incisions, and if undercorrections do occur, they are easier to correct with additional incisions (Figure 7-4).

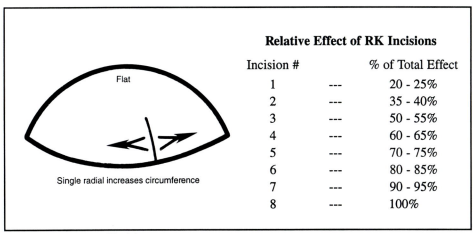

Relative Effect of RK Incisions

Incision #		% of Total Effect
1	---	20 - 25%
2	---	35 - 40%
3	---	50 - 55%
4	---	60 - 65%
5	---	70 - 75%
6	---	80 - 85%
7	---	90 - 95%
8	---	100%

Flat

Single radial increases circumference

Figure 7-4. Number of incisions.

Determining Corneal Thickness

When to Do Pachymetry

To make incisions accurately one must have correct information regarding the thickness of the cornea *in the area of the incisions*. A 500 blade depth at the beginning of a radial incision would be quite adequate for a cornea whose depth at the optical zone was 520μ but somewhat less so for an optical zone thickness of 560μ. Surgical errors, reflected in disappointing visual results, can occur when the blade extension is improperly set because of incorrect corneal depth calculations. This is not uncommon when only one "paracentral" pachymetry is done.

Pachymetry takes time and expertise. You should practice pachymetry in your office to be sure that your technique is accurate. Then if you feel more comfortable doing it in the operating room just prior to surgery you will have at least mastered the art. Your surgical results may reflect improper pachymetry either because of instrument malfunction or improper performance.

It is important that the pachymeter tip is accurately placed on the cornea and the readings repeated and verified. One reading is not adequate. You should measure the corneal thickness in every area you are going to incise. Don't just assume that because you get an "average" reading in one location that this particular cornea is "average" all over. Several studies have shown that there are thin areas in the mid-peripheral cornea in some individuals (sometimes referred to as "corneal dimples") and this thinning is not always in the infero-temporal quadrant as commonly thought.

I like to do pachymetry in my office when scheduling the case. With ultrasound pachymetry we are able to obtain a permanent printed record at the time the pachymetry is performed to aid us in our surgical planning. I find that it saves time in surgery (Figure 7-5).

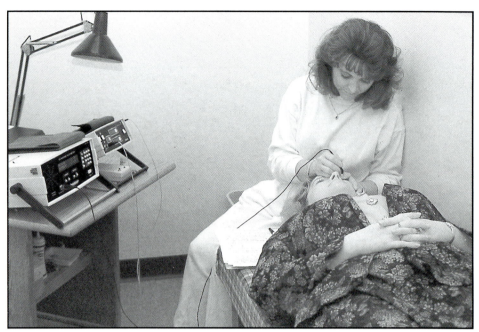

Figure 7-5. Pachymetry done in the office allows more readings and saves time in surgery.

In a long series of cases several years ago in which pachymetry was done both in the office and in the operating room, we found no significant difference in the thickness measured in the operating room as compared to the measurements taken in the office a week or two earlier. In the office the pachymetry is done under the same topical anesthesia as is used for surgery.

8

Ocular Anesthesia

The patient must be as comfortable as possible as we begin our preparation for surgery by giving Valium (diazepam) 10mg by mouth to our patients in the holding area. At this time we reinforce the previously given assurance that only eye drops and no shots will be used.

Deep Topical Anesthesia for Radial and Astigmatic Keratotomy

The patient is brought into the operating room and is made comfortable reclining in the operating chair or supine on the operating table. Prior to marking the visual axis the eye is anesthetized by repeated drops of Proparacaine (ophthaine). Here, technique is important because most of us don't realize that the usual way of instilling drops into the eye does not properly anesthetize the limbal and bulbar conjunctiva, particularly under the upper eyelid, and the patient feels the instruments (fixation ring, forceps and pressure of the diamond knife) and manipulation of the eye. The technique is as follows.

With the patient supine, the lower lid is retracted and the first drop instilled in the lower cul-de-sac (Figure 8-1). Ask the patient not to blink but to close the eyes gently. Then after ten or fifteen seconds ask the patient to look down as you lift the upper lid and place the second drop in the upper cul-de-sac. It is important to avoid putting drops directly on the pupil, thereby causing the patient to wince. This is the most important part of the technique for patient comfort. The cornea will be thoroughly washed by the anesthetic every time the patient blinks, and it is of supreme importance that the perilimbal conjunctiva be thoroughly anesthetized.

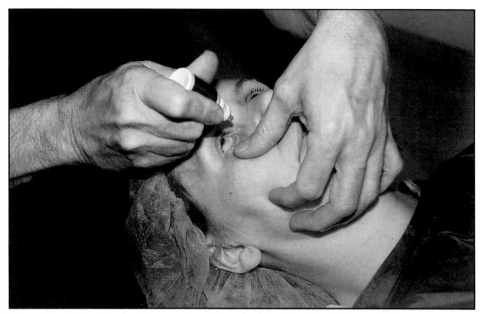

Figure 8-1. With patient looking up a drop of anesthetic is placed in the lower cul-de-sac.

Wait fifteen to twenty seconds and repeat the drop in the lower cul-de-sac with the lower lid retracted, and after another ten seconds or so retract the upper lid and place another drop in the upper cul-de-sac (Figure 8-2).

Repeat this process six or eight times as the instruments and operating room are prepared. At the conclusion of the series of anesthetic drops I mark the visual axis

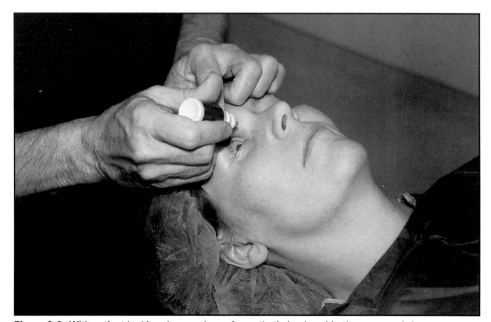

Figure 8-2. With patient looking down a drop of anesthetic is placed in the upper cul-de-sac.

under the microscope and then I scrub/gown/glove etc. while the eyelids are being prepped with Betadine (povidone iodine) in the same way you would prep for cataract surgery. I reassure the patient that all is well and use a verbal relaxation technique to allow the patient to further relax.

After the lid speculum is placed and before the optical zone is marked a drop of 4% Xylocaine (lidocaine) is instilled. This procedure takes a little more time but it is absolutely effective in preventing any sensation of pain from instrumentation during surgery. A second drop of Lidocaine is instilled at the end of the procedure for post-op comfort.

Verbal Anesthesia

After marking the center of the visual axis, and prior to prepping the eye, I use a relaxation technique sometimes referred to as *verbal anesthesia*. The patient is instructed—slowly—in a quiet voice as follows:

"Take a deep breath...now let your chest relax...now feel your back relaxing...let your stomach relax...don't tense any muscles at all...now feel your back and shoulders relaxing...let your arms totally relax, all the way to your fingertips...now feel your hips relaxing...now let your legs relax, all the way to your toes...you will feel a little like you are floating, and you will be completely at ease...just know that you are doing well, and we will let you know when we are through...we're going to wash around your eye and we'll be ready to start."

I then push away from the operating table and gown and glove while my assistant is prepping the eye. By the time I'm seated at the table the patient is usually resting quietly and completely at ease.

9

Determining the Visual Axis

A simple technique for aligning the eye on the visual axis for marking the center of the visual axis on the cornea is to place a 1mm white spot in the exact center of the objective lens of the binocular microscope directly between the right and left observer tubes. This dot, made of Liquid Paper® (used to correct typing errors), is not seen by the surgeon (the surgeon looks through the objective lens on either side of the center) but can be easily fixated by the patient looking up at the microscope. It is as if the dot is placed midway between the surgeon's eyes (Figure 9-1).

The room lights are on bright enough to easily view the eye, but the microscope light is *off*. This method does *not* depend on a light reflex or reflection of any kind. With the microscope light off the patient can easily see the objective lens of the scope and can fix on the spot in the center of the lens. The surgeon views the eye binocularly.

The body of the microscope is positioned vertically over the patient's eye so that the patient is looking straight up fixing on the center dot. The microscope light is turned off and room lights are on. The patient's fellow eye is covered and the patient told simply to "look at the dot in the center of the microscope lens" with the uncovered eye. The optical center marker is then pressed on the cornea in the center of the pupil. This apparent center of the pupil is the center of the visual axis (Figure 9-2).

This method allows the surgeon binocular visualization with three point alignment: 1) the fovea, 2) the visual axis (center of the entrance pupil), and 3) the central fixation point. No decentration or offsetting is necessary.

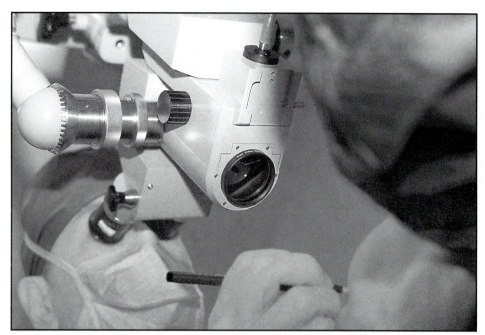

Figure 9-1. The patient looks straight up at dot in center of scope objective lens.

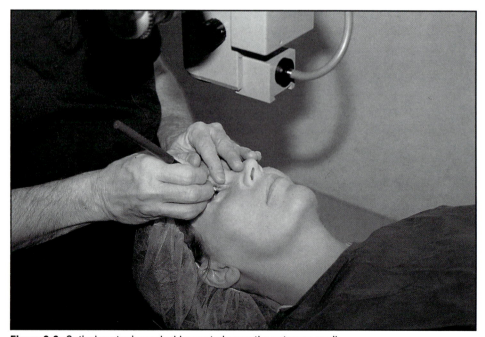

Figure 9-2. Optical center is marked by centering on the entrance pupil.

Binocularity and Stereopsis

About fifteen percent of us are not truly binocular, with varying degrees of suppression of one eye or the other. In order to use accurately the method of aligning and marking the visual axis described here you must be able to appreciate physiologic diplopia and demonstrate true binocularity.

A simple way of self testing binocularity is to hold the index finger of one hand up at arms length and bring the other index finger up at half the distance, directly in line with the distant finger. Now with both eyes open you should see one finger at distance and two fingers on either side of the distant finger. And if the fingers are aligned straight in front of you, the two "mid-distance" fingers will be of equal distance to either side of the distant finger. Now shift your gaze to the "near" finger. You should now see two distant fingers, one to each side of the near finger.

A better test of binocularity and stereopsis is the "Stare-E-O" illustrated here. To see the object illustrated, diverge your eyes as if looking at a faraway object. The two large dots will fuse, forming a third central dot. When the divergence is correct, true binocular fusion will result and slight, controlled variations in the placement of the random dots will be perceived by the brain as depth cues. An object will then appear to float above a textured background (Figure 9-3).

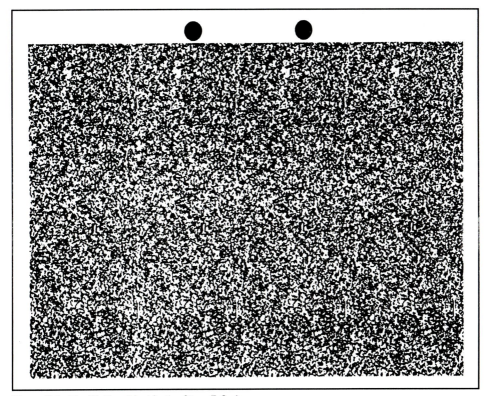

Figure 9-3. Identify the object in the Stare-E-O above.

Most methods for centering corneal surgical procedures emphasize the visual axis but do not define it properly and do not perform it accurately. Uozato and Guyton found that the best results were obtained by centering on the line of sight and center of the entrance pupil. An abstract of Uozato and Guyton's classic paper on centering the visual axis for surgical procedures is given in Appendix B.

The difficulty most surgeons have in accurately marking the visual axis is because of the traditional method of centering on a light. Corneal reflex methods of determining the visual axis may lead to optical zone decentration. The filament of most microscope lights is not coaxial and the resulting corneal reflection is decentered. When a mark is made in the "center" of the pupil with fixation on the light filament, the surgeon must decenter the mark to compensate for this decentration. Herein lies the problem. The non-lighted fixation method has been shown to be more dependable for optical zone centration since the cornea is marked at the point in line with the center of the patient's entrance pupil, performed binocularly, ignoring any corneal light reflex as explained above.

Reference

1. Thornton SP: Surgical armamentarium. In Sanders DR, Hofmann RF, and Salz JJ. (eds): *Refractive Corneal Surgery*. Thorofare, New Jersey, SLACK Inc., 1986, p. 134.

10

Astigmatic Keratotomy

Astigmatic Keratotomy Compared to Radial Keratotomy

Radial keratotomy consists of symmetrically placed corneal incisions radiating out from a central optical zone toward the limbus. These incisions increase the circumference of the peripheral cornea as they relax tissue around the circumference. This circumferential relaxation produces a stretching and flattening of the central cornea. Transverse incisions, on the other hand, are latitudinal and relax only the meridian in which they are placed. If there is no increase in the circumference of the cornea a phenomenon called *coupling* occurs. Coupling is the tendency for incisions that relax and flatten the steeper meridian to steepen the flatter meridian 90° away. The occurrence of coupling depends on the circumference of the cornea remaining essentially unchanged. The coupling effect of transverse incisions is offset or reduced by radial incisions or transverse incisions which are so long as to become semi-radial (Figures 10-1 and 10-2).

Planning Surgery with the Nomogram

This nomogram is designed as a general guide to the use of arcuate transverse incisions and will be modified by a number of variables.

Step 1: Add all the modifiers.

Step 2: Increase or decrease the amount of cylinder by the percentage determined by the modifiers.

Step 3: Use the nomogram tables for incision length and effect (Table 10-1).

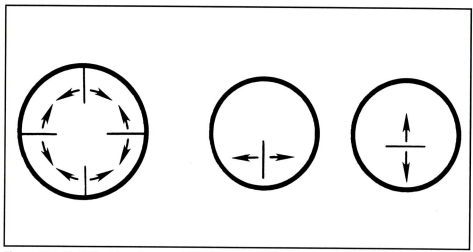

Figure 10-1. Radial incisions increase the radius of curvature circumferentially. Relaxing incisions act as if tissue is added, and the radius of curvature is increased at right angles to the incision.

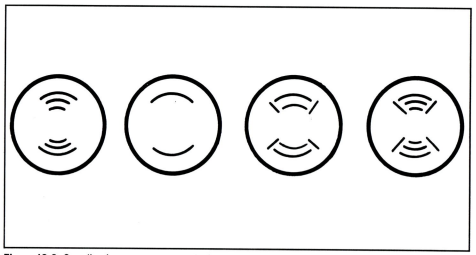

Figure 10-2. Coupling is more pronounced with several short T incisions than with one long one. Short radials outside T OZ reduce coupling 30 to 60% (depending on length) and add to meridional flattening.

A Short Cut

If you are planning both radial and transverse astigmatic incisions and have applied the modifiers to the spherical myopic component to plan the radials, you will find that about one fourth (1/4) of the amount modified for radials applies to transverse incisions. But if the case is primarily astigmatic, and you have not calculated the theoretical myopia for radial incisions, then you will need to apply the modifiers.

For example, you have calculated that your patient with an error of 4.0 - 3.0 x 90 needs (because of age, and IOP) the myopia modified by subtracting 40% to determine the *theoretical working sphere*. One fourth of this, 10%, can be subtracted from the *cylinder* without having to go through the calculation of astigmatic modifiers, and the result is -3.3 - 2.7 x 90. Note that the myopia in this case (since the cylinder is to be corrected with arcuate incisions) is the *spherical equivalent*, -5.5 diopters. -5.5 - 40% is -3.3. The cylinder does not change after calculating the spherical equivalent, and the cylinder, -3.0, can now be reduced by 10% (1/4 the amount of sphere reduction), and the *theoretical error* in this case becomes -3.3D sphere and -2.7D cylinder (see Chapter 11, *Calculating Sphere and Cylinder and Accurate Optical Zones*).

Modifiers for Astigmatic Keratotomy

All modifiers result in a percentage reduction or increase in the effect of any given amount of surgery and a change in the amount of astigmatism targeted for correction. Modifiers may increase or decrease the amount of error for any individual patient. A nomogram is then used to determine the type and amount of surgery necessary to correct this theoretical error. The tables, which are part of this nomogram, are to be referred to after calculation of the theoretical astigmatic error.

The result of surgery will vary from patient to patient depending on the patient's age, intraocular pressure and other modifiers. The modifiers must be totaled and the resulting percentage change added to or sub- tracted from the patient's astigmatic error before referring to the nomogram. The tables are then used to determine the incision length and the correction desired.

The principle patient variables with astigmatic keratotomy using arcuate transverse incisions are the amount of myopia, the amount of astigmatism, the patient's sex, age, average intraocular pressure and corneal curvature as determined by topography.

Minor modifiers include corneal thickness and any existing changes from previous surgery or injury.

The Major Variable

The most variable factor in astigmatic keratotomy is the surgeon's technique. The failure to use an accurate press-on ruler and just using estimates of incision length, the use of straight transverse rather than arcuate transverse incisions, the failure to perform pachymetry in the area of the relaxing incision and the lack of proper instrumentation all contribute to reduce predictability of the procedure.

With careful preoperative planning and proper use of state-of-the-art instrumentation, the results become more accurate and more gratifying both for the surgeon and the patient.

Table 10-1.
Thornton Nomogram for Astigmatic Keratotomy

Assumes cuts 98% deep (almost to Decemet's Membrane) along the
full length of the incision.

Age: For every year below age 30 add 1/2% to the astigmatic error. For
every year above age 30 subtract 1/2%.

Sex: In premenopausal women (under age 40) subtract three years from
actual age.

IOP: For every mm IOP below 12 add 2% to the astigmatic error. For every
mm IOP above 15, subtract 2%.

Add or subtract the sum of the modifiers (%)
from the actual amount of cylinder for the "Theoretical Cylinder."

Cylinder Corrected by Paired Arcuate Transverse Incisions

Chord Length of One Pair
Arcuate Transverse Incisions

Theoretical Cylinder	Degrees Arc
0.50 D	20°
0.75 D	23°
1.00 D	25°
1.25 D	28°
1.50 D	32°
1.75 D	35°
2.00 D	38°
2.25 D	42°
2.50 D	45°

One pair
always placed at
the 7 mm OZ

Table 10-1. (continued)
Thornton Nomogram for Astigmatic Keratotomy

Chord Length of Two Pairs
Arcuate Transverse Incisions

Theoretical Cylinder	Degrees Arc
2.00 D	23°
2.25 D	27°
2.50 D	31°
2.75 D	35°
3.00 D	39°
3.25 D	43°
3.50 D	47°
3.75 D	50°

Two pairs
outer at the 8
inner at the 6

Chord Length of Three Pairs
Arcuate Transverse Incisions

Theoretical Cylinder	Degrees Arc
3.25 D	22°
3.50 D	26°
3.75 D	30°
4.00 D	35°
4.25 D	40°
4.50 D	45°
4.75 D	50°
5.00 D	54°

Three pairs
outer just outside the 8
middle incision at the 7
inner just inside the 6

Smaller OZ (5.5 mm to 7.5 mm) -0.50 D to 1.00 D more

Astigmatic Modifiers

Age

For every year below age 30 add 1/2% to the astigmatic error. For every year above age 30 subtract 1/2% per year. Note that the age modifier for astigmatic keratotomy with transverse incisions differs from RK. This is because transverse incisions relax and flatten the cornea directly along the meridian incised as opposed to radial incisions which relax the periphery circumferentially and stretch and flatten the central cornea secondarily.

Keratometry

In the virgin cornea (unmodified by previous surgery or injury) the keratometric readings usually confirm the astigmatism detected by refraction, but manifest astigmatism is usually somewhat less than that measured by keratometry and may be partially due to lenticular astigmatism. In general, the refractive cylinder may be less than that measured by keratometry if the lenticular astigmatism is at a different axis from that in the cornea, or more if the lenticular astigmatism is in the same axis. Computer assisted corneal topography has also demonstrated that variations between refractive and keratometric cylinder may be due to irregular and asymmetric corneal curvatures (Figure 10-3).

The keratometric measurement of corneal curvature reflects curvature irregularities only in the central two or three millimeters of the cornea. Other means must be used to determine astigmatism over the entire cornea. Only computer assisted corneal topography can give information on corneal curvature outside the central 3 millimeters.

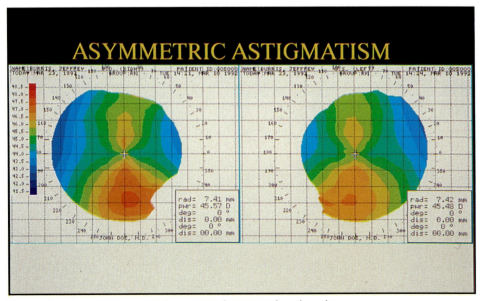

Figure 10-3. Corneal topography demonstrated asymmetric astigmatism.

Corneal Topography Analysis

Computer enhanced mapping of the corneal surface generates a color-coded contour map of the corneal surface, with power analysis easily interpreted by shades and intensity of color (Figure 10-4).

With this diagnostic device, the curvature and power of all areas of the cornea are given and analyzed, with unusual or asymmetric areas immediately apparent. In cases of asymmetric astigmatism, changes in the surgical modification of steep areas may be indicated, and asymmetric surgery may be required (Figure 10-5).

Refraction

Both manifest and cycloplegic refraction should be done! Refraction is the best measure of astigmatism in the visual axis, and in general, only the amount of astigmatism detected by refraction should be corrected. When astigmatic keratotomy is planned at the time of cataract surgery, only the keratometric or topographic cylinder should be considered since the lenticular component will be corrected by surgical removal of the lens. In postkeratoplasty cases, meaningful keratometry and refractions are sometimes impossible and it is necessary to analyze the corneal topography with a computer assisted corneal analysis system such as the EyeSys System.

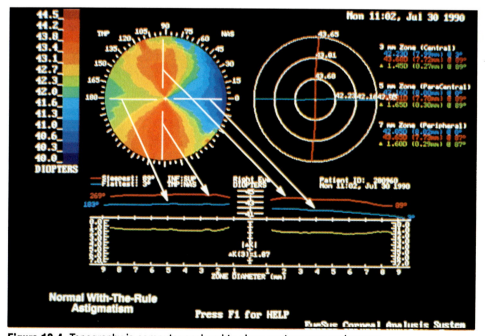

Figure 10-4. Topography is computer analyzed to show contour map and power.

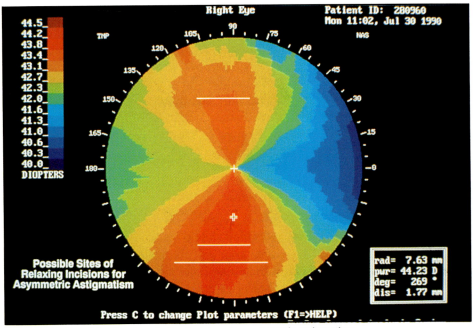

Figure 10-5. Possible sites for relaxing incisions in asymmetric astigmatism.

Intraocular Pressure

As with radial incisions, higher intraocular pressures give greater effect and lower intraocular pressures less effect. For every millimeter of mercury pressure below 12 add 2% to the astigmatic error. For every millimeter above 15 subtract 2% from the astigmatic error.

Gender and Astigmatic Incisions

In premenopausal women (under age 40) subtract three years from the actual age as hormonal differences affect tissue elasticity. This is the same for radial incisions.

Corneal Thickness

Just as with radial incisions, it appears that the thicker the cornea the greater the effect, and if the central corneal thickness is less than 490μ (0.49mm), add 10% to the astigmatic error. From 490μ to 510μ add 5%. From 580μ to 600μ subtract 5% and if the central corneal thickness is greater than 600μ, subtract 10% from the astigmatic error. Pachymetry should be performed in the area in which incisions are planned and the blade should be set so that a 95 - 98% depth is achieved along the entire length of each incision.

Depth of Incisions

Depth of incisions is not and should not be a variable. The astigmatic nomograms given with this system assume an *achieved* incision depth of 95%, i.e. almost completely through the stroma to Descemet's Membrane. An occasional microperforation only tends to confirm the adequate depth of the diamond blade micrometer setting. Technically one should make all incisions very slowly to prevent microperforations from becoming macroperforations. One should never irrigate an incision in which a microperforation has occurred.

To obtain the desired maximal depth I recommend setting the "triple-edged-arcuate" diamond blade at 100% of the pachymetry reading at the point where the incision is to be made and adjusting the depth setting in subsequent cases as determined by the effect obtained and the actual depth achieved as determined by post operative slit lamp examination.

Previous Corneal Alteration

Previous surgery affects the surgical results of astigmatic keratotomy depending on the type of the original surgery performed. Stromal scars or localized corneal thinning will affect the result with reduction of the effect in scarred or thinner areas and enhancement of the effect in thicker areas. If the central cornea has been modified, as in previous keratoplasties, more surgery must be done to achieve the effect desired, and the outcome is less predictable and more variable. If, as in most cataract procedures, only the limbus has been modified and the cornea is free from incisions or sutures, the cornea behaves more like a "virgin cornea."

Instrumentation

Reproducible precision can only be assured with proper instrumentation. I recommend the use of a 360° corneal press-on marker for measurement of precise arc-lengths at the desired optical zone. The triple-edged diamond blade design with it's 200μ square tip makes well-controlled arcuate incisions possible.

If you are limited to the wider 35-45° angled diamond blade or the tri-square diamond blade, arcuate incisions are more difficult to make and you may be forced to perform straight transverse incisions. Since the newer instruments have become available, the accuracy and reproducibility of astigmatic keratotomy has been enhanced.

Straight Versus Arcuate Transverse Incisions

It is difficult to depict a three-dimensional concept with a two-dimensional illustration and because transverse incisions have been depicted in presentations and published papers as straight lines, the potential of *coupling* has not been fully realized (Figure 10-6). All straight lines on a spherical surface are curved. Straight transverse incisions are actually inverse arcs and are therefore semi-radial, and the longer the incision the more radial it becomes. Concentric arc incisions on the other hand are parallel to the equator (truly transverse to the meridian) and therefore have greater effect on the meridian transversed.

Arcuate incisions, precisely following the curve of the circular optical zone, have the potential for greater effect because the chord length is the same as straight transverse incisions, but the actual length is about 10% longer on the curve and the entire length of the incision is at the calculated optical zone.

The difficulty in producing precise, reproducible concentric arcuate incisions has chiefly been because of instrumentation. The diamond blades used for radial and transverse corneal incisions have been relatively wide blades (either square-tipped or angled from 35° to 45°), making curved incisions difficult. The new triple-edged diamond blade design overcomes this difficulty. Still, precise arcuate incisions are difficult and require a higher degree of skill than straight. Straight incisions are easier to make.

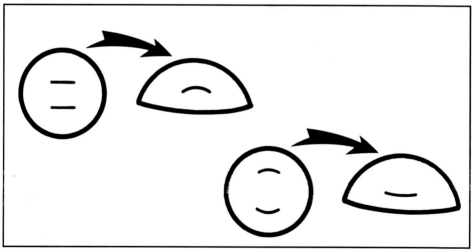

Figure 10-6. What appears to be a straight transverse line when viewed from above a spherical surface is actually an inverse arc. What appears to be a concentric arc from above is parallel to the equator and therefore transverse to the meridian.

Inverse Arc Incisions

Occasionally a patient presents with a cylinder error which, when corrected with arcuate incisions (concentric to the visual axis), will result in significant spherical myopia because of coupling. When this resulting myopia is unwanted, the traditional means of reducing it is by the use of radial incisions in addition to the arcuate ones.

With *inverse arcuate incisions*, an approach to the correction of astigmatism is possible which is minimally invasive, reduces or eliminates the need for radial incisions, requires little change in technique, and requires no special instrumentation other than that used for arcuate astigmatic incisions.

Inverse arc incisions have both transverse and radial components. They are effective because the transverse arc length is the same as concentric arc incisions but, because the ends of the incisions are at a larger optical zone, the chord length is longer. The inversely arched incision crosses the area of steep curvature, flattening it, and at the same time acts as a radial incision circumferentially because each end of the incision is virtually radial to the central visual axis.

The inverse arc incision optical zone is measured from its mid-point. It uses a modified arcuate AK Nomogram and the 360° press-on marker normally used for concentric arcuate incisions. Because the thickness of the cornea varies through a sagital distance of one half millimeter, the likelihood of microperforations during the incision is increased, and incisions must be made extremely slowly to prevent microperforations from becoming *macro*perforations. Because of its radial component it can reduce coupling up to 90%. It is minimally invasive, avoiding the need for radial incisions in most cases. Depending on age, inverse arc incisions can correct up to 5.0 diopters cylinder. Nomograms for inverse arc incisions are now available (see Appendix A).

Surgical Technique

The greatest surgical variable is the surgeon's technique. Early in the learning curve the surgeon's touch is extremely variable and, though sometimes heavy-handed, is usually more tentative in early cases and undercorrections or underresponses are more common. As in many other types of delicate surgery, there is a definite learning curve in astigmatic keratotomy. Follow the system carefully for best results.

It is good to remember that nomograms are developed by retrospective study of a large number of cases in the hands of the nomogram designer, and for comparable results the surgeon must carefully follow not only the technique advocated but also use the specific instruments recommended to achieve the desired result.

Modifier Summary for Astigmatic Correction

All modifiers result in a percentage change in the amount of astigmatism which must be targeted for correction. The modifiers must be totaled and the resulting total percentage change added to or subtracted from the patient's astigmatic error to arrive at a "theoretical error" before referring to the nomogram tables.

Example

A male age 70 with an intraocular pressure of 18 with keratometry and refraction indicating + 2.00 - 5.00 x 90.

Age 70 results in a 20% reduction (1/2% per year reduction from age 30). Intraocular pressure of 18 results in a 6% reduction for a total of 26% reduction of the actual amount of astigmatism (5.00 - 26% = 3.7 diopters "theoretical" cylinder). The nomogram indicates that two pairs of arcuate transverse incisions measuring 48° will give full correction of the 5 diopter error. A male of age thirty with the same error would obtain only 3.75 diopters correction with this same amount of surgery. Note that if straight incisions are used rather than concentric arcuate incisions, each incision would have to be longer.

Coupling

When arcuate transverse incisions are used in combination with radial incisions one must remember the law of the incised cornea which is as follows: "The change in curvature 90° away from a corneal incision is proportional to the change in the primary meridian reduced by any increase in circumference produced by radial incisions."

With the transverse incisions of astigmatic keratotomy the corneal curvature can be corrected by coupling to a sphere which is the spherical equivalent of the original error.

Using the coupling phenomenon along with modified radials, many types of astigmatism can be corrected to near plano (Figure 10-7).

Rules for Astigmatic Keratotomy Calculation and Surgical Planning

When both sphere and cylinder are to be corrected, you must determine the spherical equivalent *first*. Then apply the modifiers to the spherical equivalent (which is now considered the "spherical component"). Although the difference is not large, the most accurate correction for myopia and astigmatism is achieved by determining the spherical equivalent and *then* applying the modifiers.

The spherical equivalent for any given sphere and cylinder is the same, until age and the other modifiers are applied. However, if you apply the modifiers to the cylinder prior to determining the spherical equivalent, the chance of overcor-

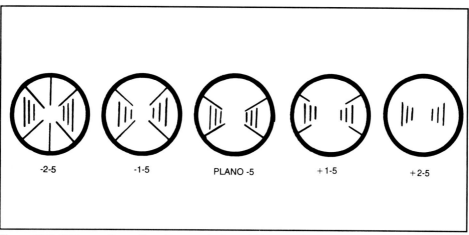

-2-5   -1-5   PLANO -5   + 1-5   + 2-5

Figure 10-7. With coupling astigmatism can be brought to near plano.

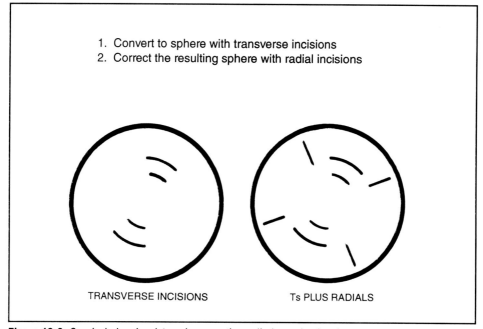

1. Convert to sphere with transverse incisions
2. Correct the resulting sphere with radial incisions

TRANSVERSE INCISIONS   Ts PLUS RADIALS

Figure 10-8. Surgical planning (steps in correcting cylinder and sphere).

recting the myopic spherical component is increased the older the patient because of the age modifier.

Both in step by step calculation and in surgical planning you should keep in mind that you want to convert the myopic sphere and cylinder error to a spherical myopia with transverse incisions *first* and then calculate the amount of correction needed with radials to correct the myopia which remains (Figure 10-8).

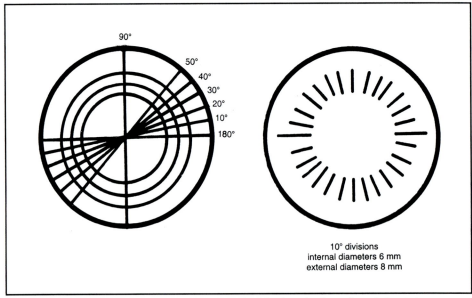

Figure 10-9. A new system for determining arcuate incision lengths for astigmatic keratotomy.

A New System for Establishing Arcuate Incision Lengths for Astigmatic Keratotomy

Whereas most previous nomograms were based on straight incisions of a given length at any of several optical zones, a new system for determining arcuate incision lengths for astigmatic keratotomy has been devised with incision lengths determined in degrees of arc at various optical zones. We are all familiar with the degrees of arc shown on refractors, phoropters and lensometers. (Figure 10-9).

Specific lengths for these arc measurements have been calculated for various optical zones (Figure 10-10).

The specific lengths required for precise and predictable astigmatism correction are now possible with instrumentation now available. With the 360° press-on corneal ruler and high magnification under the operating microscope and the new thin triple-edged-arcuate diamond blades available, very precise incisions can be made (Figures 10-11 and 10-12).

Concentric arcuate incisions are harder to make and require greater skill but the rewards of greater accuracy are worth the investment in time and energy. With perfect arcuate "T" incisions, the coupling is one to one, that is for every diopter of flattening produced in the steep meridian, there is a diopter of steepening produced in the flatter meridian 90° away.

With straight "T" incisions the coupling is reduced to about two-to-one, that is for every diopter of flattening produced in the steep meridian there is about one-half diopter steepening produced in the flatter meridian 90° away. And with inverse arc incisions, virtually all coupling can be eliminated.

Length	5mm OZ	6mm OZ	7mm OZ	8mm OZ
20°	0.9mm	1.0mm	1.2mm	1.4mm
25°	1.0mm	1.3mm	1.5mm	1.7mm
30°	1.3mm	1.5mm	1.8mm	2.0mm
35°	1.5mm	1.8mm	2.1mm	2.4mm
40°	1.7mm	2.0mm	2.4mm	2.7mm
45°	1.9mm	2.3mm	2.7mm	3.1mm
50°	2.1mm	2.5mm	2.9mm	3.4mm

Figure 10-10. Incision lengths at varying OZ.

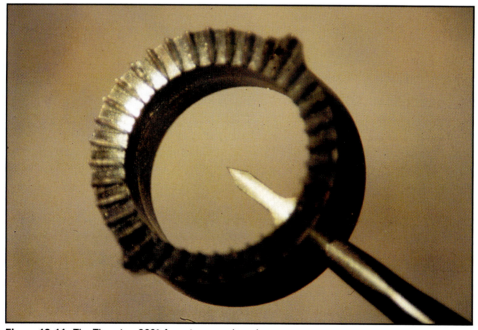

Figure 10-11. The Thornton 360° Arcuate corneal marker.

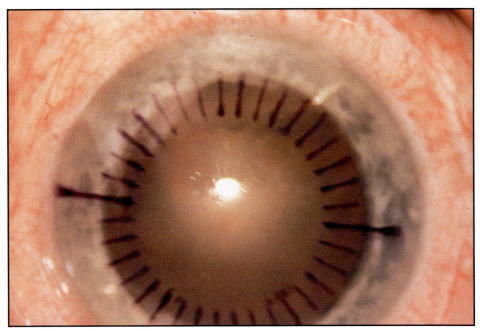

Figure 10-12. 360° Arcuate marker printed on cornea.

Summary

The nomogram used for straight transverse incisions differs from the nomogram for arcuate incisions, requiring longer straight incisions to achieve the same result as shorter arcuate incisions. Unless you use precisely the same instruments (including the Triple Edged Arcuate diamond blade and the 360° Press-on Corneal Ruler), the same approach and surgical technique, your results will not precisely duplicate those of the nomogram's originator. But as you master arcuate incisions and modify your particular surgical touch you will find your results coming very close to those given in the nomogram. And as you gain confidence in the use of arcuate incisions, you will see your efforts rewarded with greater precision.

11

Calculating Sphere and Cylinder and Accurate Optical Zones

Plus or Minus Cylinder

Both plus and minus cylinder must be used to calculate the myopia for determining optical zone size, and in both cases you must calculate the spherical equivalent if one or more diopters cylinder is present. Both forms tell you the amount of cylinder, but the minus cylinder form tells you the correct *spherical component* and helps you avoid overcorrection, and the plus cylinder form tells you the *axis of the steep meridian* and where to make T cuts.

To determine the amount of myopia for radial keratotomy incisions you must calculate the spherical component if more than 0.75 diopters cylinder is present to avoid overcorrecting the myopia and producing hyperopia (a very unwanted result) and leaving uncorrected cylinder. For example, -5 + 3 = -2 - 3. If you operated on this sphere in plus cylinder form you would overcorrect the myopia and retain the cylinder. The spherical equivalent is used for radial keratotomy calculation *only* if astigmatic keratotomy is to be performed. If the cylinder is 0.75 or less *ignore* the cylinder in your calculations. Let me emphasize this, use the spherical equivalent as the spherical component for the myopia *only if the cylinder is to be corrected by T incisions.*

You must not take any shortcuts in studying the cornea in preparation for refractive surgery. You should look at the error in both plus and minus cylinder as well as the spherical equivalent.

Calculating Plus and Minus Cylinder and Spherical Equivalent

To convert plus to minus cylinder, add the cylinder to the sphere and change the sign and axis of the cylinder by 90.°
Example: -2.00 + 3.00 x 180 = + 1.00-3.00 x 90.
To convert minus to plus, add the cylinder to the sphere and change the sign and axis of the cylinder by 90°.
Example: + 2.00 - 3.00 x 180 = -1.00 + 3.00 x 90.
To calculate the spherical equivalent, add one-half of the cylinder to the sphere.
Examples: + 2.00 - 3.00 x 180 = + 0.50 spherical equivalent.
And -2.00 + 3.00 x 180 = -0.50 spherical equivalent.

Modifying the Spherical Equivalent

If the spherical equivalent is in the plus, astigmatism *must* be corrected by arcuate transverse incisions (not straight Ts) to preserve the spherical equivalent and avoid making the patient more hyperopic.

The spherical equivalent is used as the spherical component *only when the cylinder is to be corrected.* When both sphere and cylinder are to be corrected, determine the spherical equivalent *first,* then apply the modifiers to the spherical equivalent (which is now considered the "spherical component"). Although the difference is not large, the most accurate correction for myopia and astigmatism is achieved by determining the spherical equivalent first and *then* applying the modifiers.

The spherical equivalent for any given sphere and cylinder is the same, regardless of age. However, if you apply the modifiers prior to determining the spherical equivalent, the cylinder will have more effect on the spherical equivalent as the age increases and the likelihood of overcorrecting the spherical myopia (the myopic component) is increased.

Let's look at three examples. Assume a refractive error of -4.00 -4.00 at any axis with all other variables constant.

1. At age **30** the spherical equivalent of -4.00 -4.00 is -6.00. At age 30 no modification of the sphere is necessary and the cylinder remains -4.00 and so the "theoretical error" is -6.00 -4.00.

2. At age **40** if we determine the spherical equivalent *first*, -4.00 -4.00 gives a spherical equivalent of -6.00 modified by age (-20%) which becomes 6.00 - 20% = -4.8. The cylinder of 4.00 is modified by age by -5% (one fourth the amount of radials) (4.00 - 5% = 3.8 diopters "theoretical cylinder") and the "theoretical error" becomes -4.8 -3.8.

   If however we modify the sphere and the cylinder *separately* and *then* calculate the spherical equivalent, we get -4.00 - 20% (age modifier) = 3.2 sphere, and -4.00 cyl - 5% (cylinder age modifier) = 3.8 theoretical cylinder, and the spherical equivalent then becomes 3.2 + 1.9 (one half the theoretical cylinder) = -5.1. The "theoretical error" then becomes -5.1 -3.8 and we may produce an *overcorrection* as a result.

3. At age **70** if we determine the spherical equivalent first, -4.00 - 4.00 gives a spherical equivalent of -6.00 modified by age (-60%) which becomes -2.4 diopters (-6.00 -60%) theoretical spherical component. The cylinder is modified by 20% at age 70 and 4.00 - 20% = 3.2 diopters "theoretical cylinder" and the "theoretical error" then becomes -2.4 -3.2.

   If however we modify the sphere and the cylinder *separately* and then calculate the spherical equivalent, we get -4.00 sphere -60% = 1.6 diopters sphere, and -4.00 cyl - 20% (the cylinder age modifier at age 70) = 3.2. The spherical equivalent then becomes 1.6 + 1.6 (one half the theoretical cylinder) = -3.2 "theoretical spherical equivalent" and the theoretical error becomes -3.2 -3.2 and *overcorrection is more likely.*

Avoiding Problems

To avoid overcorrections the refraction must be expressed in minus cylinder form and the spherical equivalent used in planning radial keratotomy *only* if the cylinder is to be corrected by "T" incisions. Modifiers should be applied only *after* the spherical equivalent has been determined.

The Thornton guide for both spherical and astigmatic correction is simple in theory but sometimes complex to calculate because of mathematical corrections required for age, sex, IOP and other modifiers. For this reason the nomograms for myopia and astigmatism have been programmed into several software packages which are now available.

One such program is called *Reliable Keratotomy*. This program uses the nomograms and formulas developed by myself and J.L. Gayton, MD and eliminates the need for complicated math, allowing ancillary personnel to do the calculations, much faster and more accurately than with tables and calculator, freeing the surgeon to do surgery. It is available from The Surgical Software Series, 216 Corder Road, Warner Robins, GA 31088.

Example Cases, Thornton Method of Step by Step Calculation of RK Optical Zones

All cases matched for IOP [14], CD [12], Central Pachymetry [500μ].

1. Female age 22 with spherical refraction -3.00, K 44.50. Reduce age by three years because of sex, age thus becomes 19. 30 - 19 = 11 x 2% = 22%. Add 22% to the refractive error of -3.00 diopters = -3.66 diopters. The nomogram shows that 3.66 diopters can be corrected with an optical zone of 3.75mm and eight incisions (Figure 11-1).

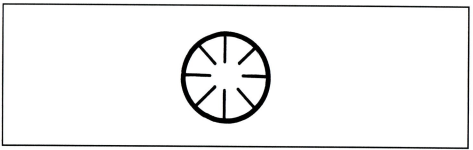

Figure 11-1. Eight radial incisions with 3.75mm OZ.

2. Female age 39 with a spherical error -3.00, K 44.50. Reduce age by three years because of sex to age 36. 6 x 2% per year reduction of effect = 12%. -3.00 - 12% = -2.64 diopters. The nomogram indicates that 2.64 diopters myopia can be corrected with an optical zone of 4.0mm with eight incisions or a 3.75mm optical zone with four incisions (Figure 11-2).

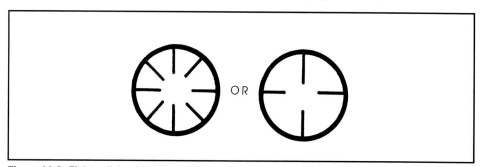

Figure 11-2. Eight radials with 4.0mm OZ or four radials with 3.75mm OZ.

3. Male age 39 with spherical refractive error of -3.00 and a K of 44.50. Age 39 (nine years over age 30) requires a reduction of the theoretical myopic error of 18%. -3.00 - 18% = -2.46 diopters. The nomogram shows that 2.46 diopters can be corrected with eight incisions at a 4.25mm optical zone or four incisions at a 4.0mm optical zone (Figure 11-3).

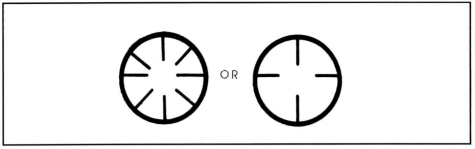

Figure 11-3. Eight radials with 4.25mm OZ or four radials with 4.0mm OZ.

4. Male age 39 with a spherical refractive error of -3.00 but with a flatter K reading of 42.50. The same percentage reduction applies in this case to give a theoretical spherical error -2.46 but because the flatter K reading is less than 42.75, the optical zone must be reduced by 0.25mm. Thus -2.46 theoretical myopic error can be corrected with eight incisions at a 4.0mm optical zone or four incisions at a 3.75mm optical zone (Figure 11-4).

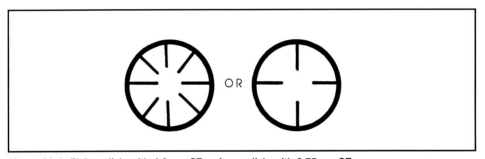

Figure 11-4. Eight radials with 4.0mm OZ or four radials with 3.75mm OZ.

5. Female age 60 with spherical refractive error of -3.00 and a K of 45.00. Age 60 -2% per year to age 50 (40%) and 1% per year from age 50 to 60 (10%) gives a 50% reduction. 50% of -3.00 = -1.5 diopters and the nomogram shows that 1.5 diopters can be corrected with four incisions at a 4.25mm optical zone (Figure 11-5).

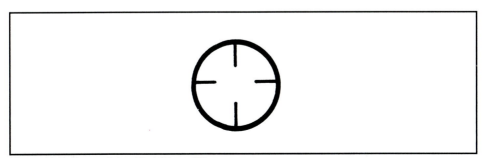

Figure 11-5. Four radials with 4.25mm OZ.

6. Female age 33 with refraction -4.00 + 0.50 x 180. Reduce age to 30 because of sex. No percentage reduction or increase is necessary at age 30 and cylinders of 0.50 to 0.75 can be ignored. The spherical component in this case is -3.50 diopters. The nomogram indicates that this error can be corrected with eight incisions at a 3.75mm optical zone (Figure 11-6).

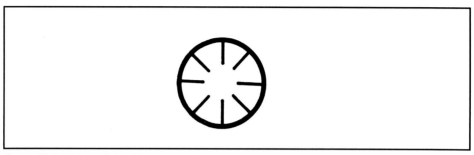

Figure 11-6. Eight radials with 3.75mm OZ.

7. Female age 33 with refraction -4.00 -0.50 x 180 and K 44.00 x 180 / 44.50 x 90. Again in this case the female sex modifier reduces the age to 30 and no percentage adjustment is necessary at age 30. Cylinders of 0.50 to 0.75 can be ignored and the spherical component of this refraction is -4.00 diopters. The nomogram indicates that this myopic error can be corrected with eight incisions with an optical zone of 3.5mm (Figure 11-7).

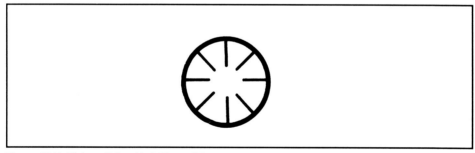

Figure 11-7. Eight radials with 3.50mm OZ.

Some Cases With More Astigmatism

(Remember the rule: The spherical equivalent is used as the *spherical component only when the cylinder is to be corrected.*)

8. Female age 25 with refraction -4.00 -2.00 x 90 and K 44.00 x 90/ 46.00 x 180. Since we are going to correct the cylinder with T incisions, we must calculate the spherical equivalent of -4.00 -2.00 which is -5.00. Reduce the age for fe-

male to 22. 30 - 22 = 8 and 8 x 2% per year = 16% increase in theoretical power. 5.00 + 16% = 5.8 diopters. The spherical equivalent has now become the myopic *spherical component* and the nomogram indicates that 5.8 diopters myopia can be corrected with eight radial incisions at a 3.0mm optical zone.

The *cylinder* requires an increase of 1/2% per year and eight years = 4% increase in cylinder and -2.00 + 4% = 2.08 diopters. The astigmatic keratotomy nomogram shows that 2.08 diopters cylinder can be corrected with one pair of arcuate transverse incisions 38° in length. Single pairs of incisions are always placed at a 7mm optical zone (Figure 11-8)

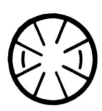

Figure 11-8. Eight radials with 3.0mm OZ and one pair of arcuates at the 7mm OZ.

9. Male age 40 with the same refraction, -4.00 -2.00 and keratometry readings of 44.00/46.00 X 180. The spherical equivalent produced by coupling is -5.00 and because of his age the reduction of the sphere power would be 20% (-5.00 -20% = -4.00 diopters). *This modified spherical equivalent now becomes the spherical component* and the nomogram indicates that a -4.00 sphere can be corrected with four radial incisions at a 3.25mm optical zone (Figure 11-9).

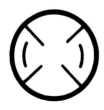

Figure 11-9. Four radials with 3.25mm OZ and one pair of arcuates at the 7mm OZ.

The cylinder is reduced only 1/2% per year from age 30, or 5% and -2.00 - 5% = - 1.9 diopters. The astigmatic keratotomy nomogram indicates that 1.9 diopters cylinder can be corrected with one pair of arcuate transverse incisions 38° in length.

Case Histories

Case One

A 33 year old woman presenting with difficulty wearing contact lenses because of recurrent irritation and scratched corneas. Dry eyes have been a problem. Refraction: OD -4.00 -0.25 x 90, OS -5.00 sphere. Both eyes correct to 20/25. IOP 10 OU, CD 12mm OU, CP (central pachymetry) OD 486 & OS 494. At age 33 the ideal result would be to leave the patient slightly myopic.

Solution: Sex reduced theoretical age to 30. Intraocular pressure of 10 increased the myopia by +4% CP of 486 increased the theoretical myopia in the right eye by 10% and CP of 494 increased the theoretical myopia in the left eye by 5%. (Rule: for Central Pachymetry less than 490, add 10% to the myopia. From 490 to 510, add 5%. From 510 to 580 make no change. For CP 580 to 600, subtract 5%, and above 600 subtract 10% from the myopia.) The net change in the theoretical power in the right eye was +14% and in the left eye +9%.

The left eye, with a theoretical myopia of -5.45, was operated on first with a 3.0mm optical zone and eight radial incisions carried from the optical zone to the limbus at a depth of 530 microns (98% deep at the 3mm optical zone) The right eye, with a theoretical myopia of -4.56, was operated on three months later with a 3.25mm optical zone and eight radial incisions carried from the optical zone to the limbus at a depth of 530 microns (98% deep at the 3.25mm optical zone) (Figure 11-10).

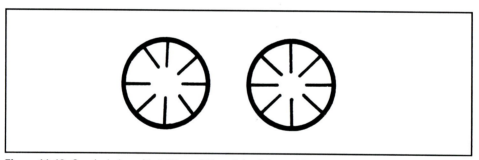

Figure 11-10. Surgical plan with 3.25mm OZ on right, 3.0mm OZ on left.

At the six month examination her vision was 20/20- in both eyes without correction and refraction showed her to have -0.50 sphere in both eyes.

Case Two

A 30 year old woman with progressive myopia and astigmatism and complaints of headaches and dry eyes. She had difficulty working at her computer. Sixteen months prior to our first examination her ophthalmologist prescribed OD -4.75 -0.50 x 30 and OS -6.25 sphere. On cycloplegic refraction she was found to have OD -5.25 -0.75 x 20 and OS -6.25 -0.75 x 165. She corrected to 20/25 in both eyes.

IOP measured 12mm Hg in both eyes and her central pachymetry was 588 OD and 584 OS. CD was 11.8 OU.

Solution: With apparent increase in her myopia and astigmatism which had not previously been corrected, it was deemed wise to plan for a slight undercorrection of her myopia without directly addressing the astigmatism. Female sex reduced theoretical age to 27 for a 6% increase in her myopia. Central pachymetry of 588 OD and 584 OS reduced it 5% , for a net change of + 1%. Her theoretical myopia became OD -5.30 and OS -6.31.

The left eye was operated on first with a 3.0mm optical zone and eight radial incisions carried from the optical zone to the limbus at a depth of 625 microns (98% deep at the 3mm optical zone) and deepened to 665 microns from the 5mm optical zone. There were no microperforations. Two months later her right eye had a similar procedure with a 3mm optical zone and eight radial incisions at a depth of 625 microns, without redeepening (Figure 11-11).

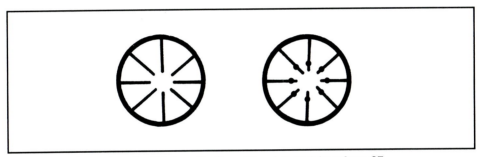

Figure 11-11. Deepening of radials from the 5mm OZ on left. Both have 3mm OZ.

Three months after the second eye surgery her uncorrected vision was 20/40 on the right and 20/50 on the left and she corrected to 20/25 in both eyes with OD -0.25 -0.50 x 20 and OS -0.50 -0.50 x 165.

Case Three

A 26 year old woman presented with glasses showing a refraction of OD -2.25 -1.50 x 98 and OS -2.00 -1.25 x 75. On cycloplegic refraction she was found to have OD -1.75 -1.75 x 100 and OS -1.50 -1.75 x 70 correcting to 20/20 in both eyes. She complained of dry eyes and discomfort with contact lenses. Keratometry showed OD 4712 x 35 / 4650 x 130 and OS 4637 x 40 / 4700 x 135. CD 11.8 OU, IOP 16 OU and central pachymetry OD 529,OS 533.

Solution: Because her job required close work we set out to undercorrect her by 0.75 to one diopter. Since we plan to correct her astigmatism, the first step is to calculate the spherical equivalent. The spherical equivalent OD is -1.75 x 1/2 = 0.87 + 1.75 = 2.62 and OS 0.87 + 1.50 = 2.37. Female age 26 is reduced to 23 for a 14% increase in theoretical myopia and IOP of 16 reduces it 2% for a net increase of 12% for myopia, and her theoretical myopia becomes OD 2.62 + 12%

= 2.93 and OS 2.37 + 12% = 2.65. Because astigmatism is changed only 1/2% per year the amount of increase in her theoretical astigmatism is only 1.5% (1.75 + 1.5% = 1.77) Her theoretical myopia becomes OD -2.93 - 1.77 and OS became -2.37 - 1.77. The right eye now has a theoretical myopia of -2.93 and the left eye -2.37 because of coupling resulting when the astigmatism is corrected with T incisions.

The non-dominant left eye was operated on first with a 4.25mm optical zone (remember, we're deliberately undercorrecting) with four radial incisions at 98% depth at the optical zone and one pair of 32° long arcuate incisions across the 140° meridian. One month later she underwent a similar procedure in the right eye with 4.25mm optical zone and four radials at a depth of 600 microns with one pair of 32° long arcuate incisions at a 7mm optical zone across the 20° meridian (Figure 11-12).

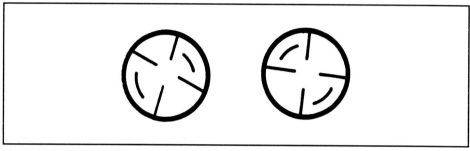

Figure 11-12. Surgical plan combining radials with arcuates.

At her two-month post-op examination her uncorrected vision was 20/30-2 on the right and 20/30 on the left corrected to 20/20 OU with a refraction of OD -0.75 -0.50 X 100 and OS -0.50 sphere. The patient stated that she was quite comfortable with this slight undercorrection.

Case Four
A 49 year old male with history of inability to wear contact lenses because of "unusual astigmatism." Both manifest and cycloplegic refraction revealed OD -5.50 -2.00 x 10 (-7.50 + 2.00 x 100) correcting to 20/25 -2 and OS -4.75 -0.25 x 90 correcting to 20/25. IOP 14 OU, CD 12 OU, CP (central pachymetry) OD 528, OS 534, and Ks verified the refractive cylinder.

Solution: Because of the patient's age and anisometropia he was advised that "monovision" would be targeted, leaving the right eye more myopic. Since we are correcting the cylinder with T incisions we must first determine the spherical equivalent. The spherical equivalent (-5.50 -2.00 = S E 6.50) now becomes the *spherical component*. Age 49 reduces his myopia by 38% and his astigmatism by 9.5%. In the right eye -6.50 -38% = -4.03 for the spherical component and 2 - 9.5% = -1.81 for the cylinder. The modified spherical equivalent, -4.03 (since we are correcting the cylinder with T incisions) now becomes the "working" spherical component.

The right eye was operated on first using a 3.25mm optical zone with four radials 98% deep at the 3.25mm optical zone. Because corneal topography showed more than 75% of the steepness in the 90 - 100° meridian to be in the upper semi-meridian, one pair of arcuate incisions were placed at the 7mm optical zone 98% deep (at that point) with the length of the incision 35° above and 20° below.

One month post-op his vision OD was 20/50 uncorrected, correcting to 20/25 with -1.25 -0.50 x 15. Seven weeks after the first procedure RK was performed on the left eye with a 3.75mm optical zone and four radial incisions at a depth of 665 microns (98% deep at the 3.75mm optical zone) (Figure 11-13).

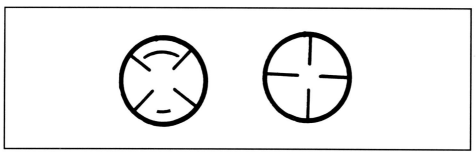

Figure 11-13. Surgical plan with asymmetric arcuate incisions in right cornea.

The two month post-op exam showed uncorrected vision of 20/50 on the right and 20/25 on the left with refraction of OD -1.50 -0.25 and OS -0.25 sphere.

Case Five

A 47 year old woman with history of difficulty wearing contact lenses because of "frequent infections." Her referring ophthalmologist confirmed that she had a superficial corneal ulcer in the left eye several years ago. She was correctable to 20/25-2 in both eyes with OD -2.00 -1.50 x 5 and OS -2.00 - 1.00 x 5. IOP measured 10 OD and 12 OS. CD 12 OU. Central pachymetry 484 OD and 482 OS. Ks OD 42.75 x 172 / 43.87 x 82 and OS 42.37 x 3 / 42.75 x 92.

Solution: Age 47 requires a reduction of 34% of her myopia (47 - 30 = 17 x 2 = 34) and 8.5% reduction of the cylinder (1/2% per year). Her IOP of 10 requires a reduction of 4% (2% per mm below 12). Her central pachymetry of 484 and 482 requires that 10% be added to her myopia.

Since we are going to correct her cylinder with T incisions we begin by determining the spherical equivalent (-2.75) This spherical equivalent (now the *spherical component*) is now modified by age (-34%), IOP (-4%) and corneal thickness (+ 10%) for a net reduction of -28%. Thus her theoretical "working" myopic error for her right eye becomes -1.98 (2.75 - 28%) and the cylinder becomes 1.37 (1.5 - 8.5%). The nomogram indicates that 1.98 D myopia can be corrected with four radials from a 4.25mm optical zone and 1.37 D cyl can be corrected with one pair of arcuate T incisions 28° long at the 7mm optical zone.

The right eye underwent radial keratotomy and astigmatic keratotomy with four radials carried 98% deep from the 4.25mm optical zone to the limbus and one pair of arcuate T incisions 28° long at the 7mm optical zone across the 95° meridian. The incision depth was 580 microns. Two months post-op her vision was 20/25 uncorrected with a plano sphere refraction. Ten weeks after the first procedure the left eye underwent radial keratotomy with four radial incisions from the 4.25mm optical zone 98% deep at the optical zone with one pair of 23° long arcuate T incisions across the 95° meridian (Figure 11-14).

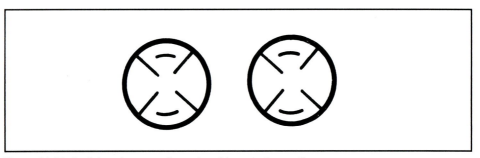

Figure 11-14. Radials reduce myopia produced by arcuate coupling.

At the six-month examination her uncorrected vision was OD 20/30 and OS 20/25-3 corrected to 20/20 with -0.50 sphere and -0.75 sphere.

Case Six

A 43 year old woman presented with inability to wear either hard or soft contact lenses stating that her eyes stayed dry and "contacts were always uncomfortable." Finger-counting vision could be corrected to 20/25 with OD -6.00 -0.50 x 45 and OS -5.25 -1.25 x 165. IOP was 12mm Hg in both eyes, CD 11mm, Central Pach OD 567, OS 547, and topography confirmed the symmetrical oblique astigmatism.

Solution: Women are considered pre-menopausal to age 40 so her age would not need to be reduced because of sex. Thus her age requires a reduction of power of 26% (43-30 = 13 x 2 = 26%). The 11mm corneal diameter requires an increase of 0.25 D to the power so OD -6.00 + 0.25 = -6.25 - 26% = -4.62D, and because of minimal astigmatism (0.50D) in the right eye, no astigmatic correction was planned for that eye.

The left eye had 1.25D cylinder and so for the left eye the first step is to determine the spherical equivalent (-5.25 -1.25 = SE -5.87) plus 0.25 because of the 11mm corneal diameter = 6.12. Less 26% = -4.52 and the cylinder is reduced 6% (1/2% per year x 13 years) and 1.25 -6% = 1.2 D. The nomogram tells us that 4.52 diopters myopia can be corrected with four radials with an optical zone of 3mm, and 1.2D cylinder can be corrected with a pair of 25° long arcuate transverse incisions.

RK and AK were first performed on the left eye as determined by the nomogram (four radials from a 3mm optical zone, and one pair of arcuate T incisions 25° long at the 7mm optical zone) with the arcuate incisions 95% deep across the 75° meridian.

At one week her uncorrected vision was 20/50 with a refraction of OS -1.75 sphere. One month after the first procedure, because of the apparent undercorrection in the left eye, she underwent RK in the *right* eye with a 3.25mm optical zone and eight radial incisions carried from the optical zone to the limbus at 98% depth at the optical zone (Figure 11-15).

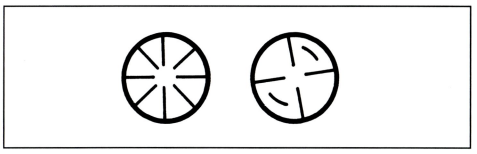

Figure 11-15. Response of left eye helped in planning surgery for right eye.

One week later her refraction was OD -0.75 sphere and OS -3.25 sphere. At the three-month examination her uncorrected vision was OD 20/25 and OS 20/200 with a refraction in the left eye of -2.75 sphere.

An enhancement procedure was performed in the left eye four months after the original procedure using a 3mm optical zone with four additional radial incisions at a 98% depth. The radials skipped the previously placed arcuate incisions (Figure 11-16).

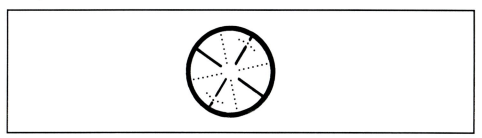

Figure 11-16. Surgical plan for enhancement, avoiding previous incisions.

One month following enhancement surgery the left eye refracted -1.00 -0.50 x 165 with uncorrected vision of 20/60. The right eye remained -0.75 sphere with uncorrected vision of 20/25. Because of the relatively high myopic error initially the patient had been advised that full correction should not be anticipated and, despite enhancement surgery, about one diopter myopia remained. This patient requires glasses for distance vision and corrects to 20/25 OU. This case illustrates the probable presence of unforeseen biological variables.

12

Thornton Method for Achieving High Power Corrections

When you determine that the working sphere is 5.00 diopters or more you note that the range of myopic power that can be corrected with any given optical zone varies increasingly as the target power or "working sphere" increases. This is an indication of the increased variability of the results of incisional surgery in higher degrees of myopia and it is in this range of powers that the surgeon's skill is the determinant of the precise amount of correction achieved.

It is logical to ask how you would get predictable correction of 5.25 diopters in one eye with a 3.0 mm optical zone and a correction of 6.0 diopters in another eye with the same sized optical zone, and one answer is in maximal extension of the blade and the amount of pressure you exert on the diamond knife with each incision for greater depth in eyes with greater myopia. This is a technique that one learns with practice.

Also, to get more effect, you want to make the deep incisions as long as possible short of crossing the limbus. And so, using the American 35° blade, when the incision is completed to the limbus, you remove the blade and turn it around and reinsert it at the limbus at the end of the incision and "square up" the incision by bringing the knife back a couple of millimeters in the outer end of the incision, without extending the blade to "redeepen."

To achieve even higher corrections, redeepening of the incisions with increased blade length is necessary from either or both the 5 and the 7mm optical zones (see nomogram in Appendix A). Slightly higher corrections may result by deepening from the 8mm optical zone but *not* from the 9mm optical zone or beyond to avoid cutting *too deep* in the extreme periphery.

When you want to achieve a higher correction of myopia, the nomogram provides a guide, but the surgeon with experience learns to modify the outcome by his touch. Correction of higher degrees of myopia should not be attempted until you have gained experience with lower powers.

Titration for Greater Precision

Secondary Optical Zones

The basic Thornton RK Nomogram (see Chapter 4) gives a range of power with each optical zone and leaves some latitude within that range for variable response to the surgery. It is possible for the surgeon, with careful planning and attention to technique, to further determine the amount of response. This response can be titrated in several ways. The main two are by "squaring up" the ends of each incision and by deepening the incisions at any of several optical zones.

Squaring Up

Squaring up the ends of the incisions in the periphery assures that the amount corrected will be in the desired range for the amount targeted in the nomogram. If that amount is just barely into that range, you can increase the effect of the incisions from a *secondary* optical zone, the amount of increased effect determined by the size of the secondary optical zone.

Redeepening

Since deepening (redeepening) produces a "step" at the base of the incision from the point redeepened, and this step may diffract light and produce glare, it is best to keep the secondary optical zone outside the range of the normally dilated pupil, and the 5mm optical zone is usually the smallest secondary optical zone recommended.

By utilizing the 5 and the 7mm secondary optical zones, the surgeon can *titrate* and increase incrementally the effect of incisions from any given primary optical zone. Redeepening all incisions 95 to 98% depth from the 7mm optical zone with a 4 or 8 radial pattern will give an increase in effect of approximately 5%, or about 0.50D. Redeepening 95 to 98% depth from the 5mm optical zone will give an increased effect of approximately 10%, or about 0.75D. Redeepening to 98% from *both* the 5 and the 7mm optical zone will give an increased effect of from 1 to 1.25D, or about 15% additional effect.

Avoiding Progressive Hyperopia

One of the factors thought to be involved in "progressive hyperopia" is incisions carried too deep in the extreme periphery, leaving not enough stroma to support the corneal circumference. It is in this extreme periphery that the deep stromal tissue assumes a circumferential pattern, the "Ligamentum circulare" or "ligament of Kokott." If this deep tissue is cut there is no restraining structure to oppose the continued increase of corneal "expansion" and the corneal circumference may continue to increase with stimuli such as increased IOP, rubbing the eye, external pressures on the eye during sleep, etc. The inevitable result is increased stretch on the central cornea and increased flattening centrally over time.

I recommend deepening of incisions from optical zones well away from the extreme periphery and, except in cases where I want to get *maximal* effect, I deepen from the 5 or the 7mm optical zones.

In cases where I have more than 7.5 diopters myopia to correct I will use eight incisions redeepened at the 5 *and* the 7mm optical zone with the blade fully extended to get an *achieved* depth of 98% in the area of both the 5 and 7mm optical zone. To do this I usually have to set my blade at 100% of the pachymetry reading *at the point at which I begin redeepening*. In confirmation of the fact that I am adequately deep I get microperforations in more than 20 percent of cases in which I am redeepening for maximal effect.

I reserve "sequential" redeepening (deepening from the 5, the 7 *and* the 8 millimeter optical zones) for those cases of from 8 to 10 diopters myopia, and use 16 radial incisions in the primary procedure only in those cases of 10 diopters or more.

Another factor which some feel contributes to progressive hyperopia, and possibly irregular astigmatism as well, is inclusions in radial incisions. These inclusions of cellular debris, whether blood or epithelial cells, become microcystic and may later need to be removed. For this reason I recommend irrigation of any incision containing visible inclusions of blood or other cellular debris at the end of the procedure.

13

Computer Assisted Corneal Topography

Corneal topography is a powerful new diagnostic tool that has become invaluable in cataract and refractive surgery. Corneal topography, sometimes referred to as computer assisted videokeratography, or CAVK, is rapidly becoming the standard by which ophthalmologists determine the shape, and sometimes the health, of patients' corneas. Irregular, asymmetric and occult pathologic astigmatism are diagnosable more accurately with corneal topography than by any other means.

The color-coded corneal contour map provided by the EyeSys topography system provides information that is easy to relate to the refractive and anatomic characteristics of the eye. It is based on the familiar Placido technology, but provides measurements on nearly 6,000 separate points with the warm colors (reds, orange and yellows) indicating steep areas and cool colors (greens, blues and violets) indicating flatter areas.

Keratometry, with its measurement of only four points on the cornea, with averaging of the two principal meridians, cannot possibly give all of the information needed to perform modern refractive surgery. These systems have been shown to be ideal in helping to predict the best therapeutic approaches in several problem areas such as post-operative management of penetrating kerato-plasty and IOL calculations in irregular corneas.

Nomograms for astigmatic keratometry had to be modified with the discovery of occult asymmetric astigmatism. In cases of asymmetry, the greatest surgical effect is obtained by placing the incisions in the steeper areas as indicated by topography.

Asymmetry

When there is significant asymmetry in the astigmatism as shown by topography, the incisional correction should be modified to prevent unforeseen surprises and undesirable results.

If the nomogram calls for two pairs of arcuate incisions 25° in length, the total incisional length is 50° on each side or 100° total. This total incisional length can be redistributed into segments to fit the asymmetric need as indicated by topography. If 75% of the steepness is on one side (in one semimeridian) you can move 75% of the total incisional length to that semimeridian and the resulting correction would be two 37° incisions in the steeper semimeridian (one 37° long arcuate incision at the 6mm optical zone and one 37° arcuate incision at the 8mm optical zone), and one 25° long incision on the 7mm optical zone in the less steep side or semimeridian (Figure 13-1).

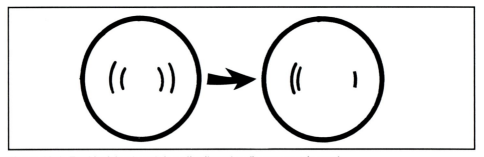

Figure 13-1. Total incision length is redistributed to fit asymmetric need.

Redistribution of Arcuate Incisions

If the calculated length of the incision exceeds the area of steepness as shown by corneal topography, the long incision may be divided into additional incisions. For example, if the nomogram suggests one pair of arcuate incisions with an incision length of 45° and the topography indicated that the steep area covers only 35,° that incision can be converted into a pair of 23° long incisions. All single pairs of incisions are placed at a 7mm optical zone. So, if a single incision is divided into two shorter incisions, these incisions would be placed at the 6mm and 8mm optical zones (Figure 13-2).

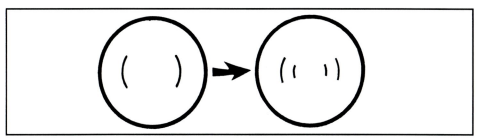

Figure 13-2. Long incisions may be divided into shorter incisions.

Axis Variation by Topography

If your calculations indicate that you have 3.25D of cylinder by keratometry at 20° and the topography picture (computer assisted videokeratography map) shows the majority of the steepness in the 50° meridian, you must modify the placement of your incisions *as determined by topography*. Axis modification is indicated with any variation of 15° or more between the refractive/keratometric and the topographic axis.

We have learned that keratometry (which measures only four points on the cornea near the optical zone) is an indication of the corneal curvature in the central 2mm but is modified by the curvature of the peripheral cornea and may not reflect the true source of the astigmatism.

The nomogram for arcuate astigmatic keratotomy incisions indicates that 3.25D cylinder can be corrected by two *pairs* of arcuate incisions 43° in length (i.e., one incision 43° in length on each side of the cornea at the 6mm optical zone and one incision 43° in length on each side of the cornea at the 8mm optical zone).

If the axis by topography is significantly different from keratometry as in this example, the altered axis must be figured in your surgical plan. If the majority of the steepness in the peripheral cornea is *outside* the 7mm optical zone, the incisions must be placed nearer the meridian indicated by topography (Figure 13-3).

If the area of steepness extends *nearer* to the center than the 6mm optical zone, the incisions should be placed nearer to the meridian indicated by the *refraction* and *keratometry* because it is this steep area that is causing the astigmatism in the central visual axis (Figure 13-4).

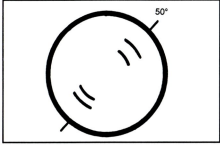

Figure 13-3. Incision placement modified when topography differs from keratometry.

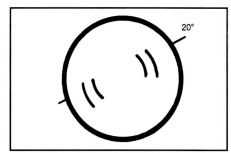

Figure 13-4. Central steepness corrected by incisions on refractive axis.

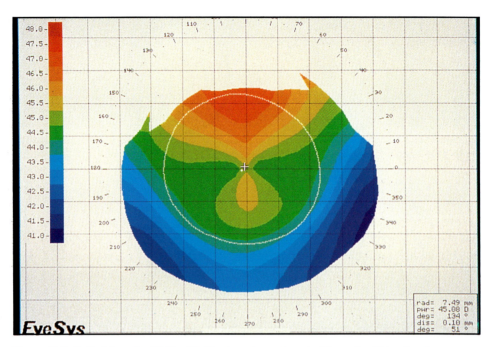

Figure 13-5. Patient A, male, 47. The "hot" colors show where incisions should be placed.

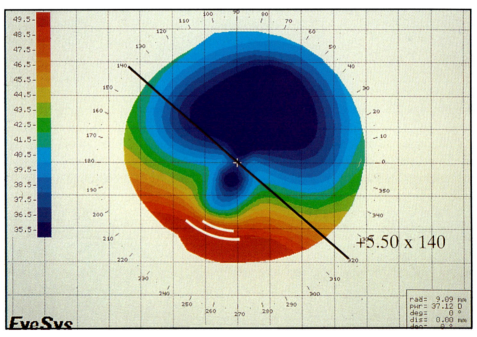

Figure 13-6. Patient B, female, 33. Topography shows where incisions should be placed—well away from misleading refractive axis.

Asymmetry in Addition to Axis Alteration

If, in addition to the axis shift, the astigmatism is asymmetrical, the relative amount of steepness on each side must be figured in also.

Because of these multiple factors influencing the placement, length and configuration of astigmatic incisions, many refractive surgeons are depending on computer programs to assist them in the determination of their corrective procedures. Computer software programs are available to aid both in proper axis determination and any necessary redistribution of arcuate incisions.

The basic principles of redistribution of incisions (i.e., the total length of the incision being redistributed as suggested by topography) remain the same when the axis is altered. In fact, the topographic picture frequently tells you the location of "hot" colors, where to place the incisions, and, by the area *covered* by the hot colors, the allowable length of these incisions.

14

Inverse Arc Incisions

A New Approach to the Correction of Astigmatism

With coupling, arcuate transverse corneal relaxing incisions flatten the meridian incised and steepen the meridian 90° away. In this chapter we demonstrate a new method of correcting steep corneal curvature without inducing coupling, by utilizing both transverse and radial components of the same incision. This technique has been found useful in cases of myopic astigmatism in which reduction of the myopic spherical equivalent, otherwise produced by arcuate incisions, is possible without having to place additional radial incisions.

Occasionally a patient presents with a cylinder error which, when corrected with arcuate incisions, will result in significant spherical myopia because of coupling. For example, a plano -4.00 diopter cylinder error, when corrected with arcuate incisions, will produce a resulting -2.00 diopter spherical error because of one-to-one coupling. When this resulting myopia is unwanted, the traditional means of reducing it is by the use of radial incisions in addition to the arcuate ones (Figure 14-1). *Inverse arcuate incisions* are a new approach to the correction of astigmatism which are minimally invasive, eliminate or reduce the need for radial incisions, require little change in technique, and require no special instrumentation other than that used currently for arcuate astigmatic incisions.

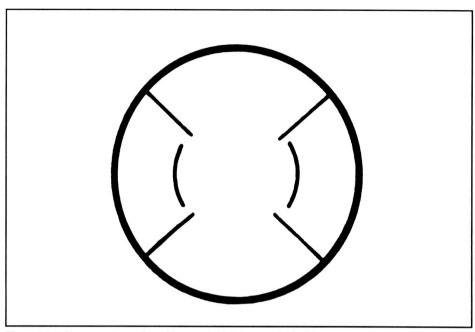

Figure 14-1. Because of coupling with arcuate incisions, radial incisions are needed to reduce myopia.

Inverse arc incisions have both transverse and radial components (Figure 14-2). They work because the transverse length in degrees of arc is the same as concentric arc incisions though the chord length is longer. For example, a concentric arc incision of 35° has a chord length of 2.3mm at a 7mm optical zone, whereas an inverse arc of 35,° with its ends at the 8mm optical zone and its mid-point at the 7mm optical zone, has a chord length of 2.6mm. The inversely arced incision crosses the area of steep curvature, flattening it, and at the same time acts as a radial incision circumferentially, because each end of the incision is virtually radial to the central visual axis.

The inverse arc incision optical zone is measured from its midpoint. It uses a modified Arcuate AK Nomogram and the 360° press-on ruler normally used for concentric arcuate incisions. Because the thickness of the cornea varies through a saggital distance of one half millimeter (from the 8 to the 7mm optical zone), the incisions must be made extremely slowly to prevent microperforations from becoming macroperforations. Because of its radial component it can reduce coupling up to 90%. It is minimally invasive, avoiding the need for radial incisions in most cases. Depending on age, inverse arcuate incisions can correct up to 5.0 diopters cylinder (Table 14-1).

Table 14-1.
Thornton Nomogram for Astigmatic Keratotomy
with Inverse Arcuate Incisions

Assumes cuts 98% deep (almost to Descemet's Membrane) along the full length of the incision.

Age: For every year below 30 add 1/2% to the astigmatic error. For every year above age 30 subtract 1/2%.

Sex: In pre-menopausal women (under age 40) subtract three years from actual age.

IOP: For every mm IOP below 12 add 2% to the astigmatic error. For every mm IOP above 15, subtract 2%.

Add or subtract the sum of the modifiers (%) from the actual amount of cylinder for the "Theoretical Cylinder."

Inverse arc incisions, because of their transverse *and* radial components, *cancel out any potential coupling* but retain their meridional flattening potential because their arc length is based on established concentric arcuate incision lengths (the Thornton Astigmatic Keratotomy Nomograms).

The optical zones given are for the *mid-point* of the inverse arc. Single pairs of incisions are always placed mid-point at the 7 mm OZ. Double pairs of incisions are always placed mid-point on the 6 and 7 mm OZ, and three pairs are always placed with the mid-point of the inner pair just inside the 6 mm OZ, the middle pair placed mid-point on the 7 mm OZ and the third, outer, pair placed mid-point just touching outside the 8 mm OZ.

Table 14-1. (continued)
Thornton Nomogram for Astigmatic Keratotomy
with Inverse Arcuate Incisions

Cylinder Corrected by Paired Inverse Arcuate Incisions

Chord Length of One Pair
Inverse Arcuate Incisions
Theoretical

Cylinder	Degrees Arc
1.00 D	25°
1.25 D	28°
1.50 D	32°
1.75 D	35°
2.00 D	38°
2.25 D	42°
2.50 D	45°

Chord Length of Two Pairs
Inverse Arcuate Incisions
Theoretical

Cylinder	Degrees Arc
2.00 D	23°
2.25 D	27°
2.50 D	31°
2.75 D	35°
3.00 D	39°
3.25 D	43°
3.50 D	47°
3.75 D	50°

Chord Length of Three Pairs
Inverse Arcuate Incisions
Theoretical

Cylinder	Degrees Arc
3.25 D	22°
3.50 D	26°
3.75 D	30°
4.00 D	35°
4.25 D	40°
4.50 D	45°
4.75 D	50°
5.00 D	54°

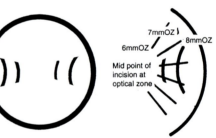

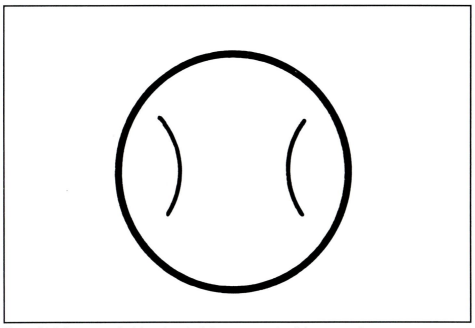

Figure 14-2. Inverse arc incisions have both transverse and radial components.

A Representative Case

A 66 year old man was referred because of bothersome astigmatic anisometropia with a history of cataract surgery with lens implantation a year or so previously. The left eye presented with a refraction of -0.25 -0.25 x 85, and uncorrected vision of 20/20. The right eye had achieved a post-operative refraction of plano -2.50 x 100, correcting to 20/20, but with an uncorrected vision of 20/50-.

Because of his desire for improved uncorrected vision at distance to match that of the fellow eye, arcuate corneal relaxing incisions (transverse incisions concentric to the visual axis) were considered. Allowing for his age and other modifiers the arcuate incisions would have been 35° in length, and because of the one-to-one coupling obtained with accurately placed arcuate incisions, he would have ended up with about -1.25 diopters spherical myopia, requiring four radial incisions to reduce the myopia.

To reduce the cylinder by about 2.00 diopters and reduce the spherical myopia produced by coupling without having to place radial incisions, paired incisions of 35° length (as determined by the AK Arcuate Nomogram) were planned as *inverse arcs* (Figure 14-3), measured by the 360° press-on corneal ruler (Figure 14-4).

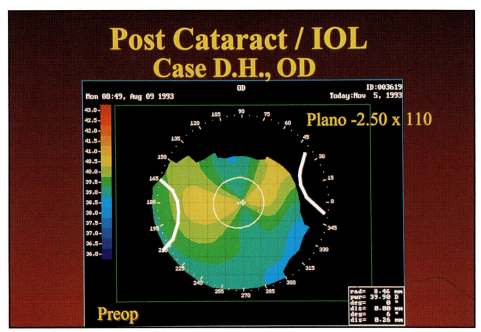

Figure 14-3. Inverse arcuate incisions.

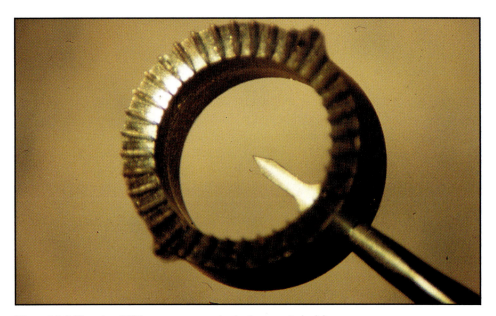

Figure 14-4. Thornton 360° press-on corneal ruler for arcuate incisions.

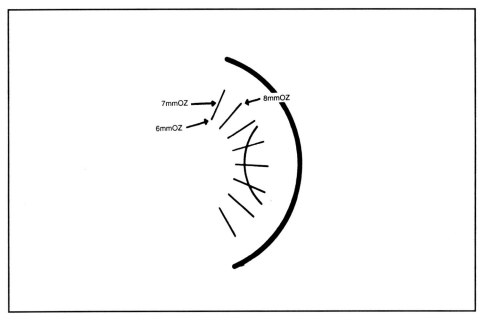

Figure 14-5. The central point of single inverse arc incisions is at the 7mm OZ.

The Surgical Plan

To correct the cylinder (2.00D, reduced by age and other modifiers to 1.75D "theoretical cylinder") the Arcuate AK Nomogram calls for a pair of concentric arcuate incisions 35° in length across the steep meridian at the 7mm optical zone. For inverse arcs the same recommended length (35°) was used but the incisions began at the 8mm optical zone and the central point of the incisions at the 7mm optical zone (Figure 14-5), for a saggital inverse section height of 0.5mm. The inverse arcs served both to relax the tissue across the steep meridian (reducing the cylinder) and at the same time relax the corneal periphery, increasing the circumference and reducing the myopic sphere.

The 360° press-on corneal ruler was applied to the cornea, centered on the visual axis, and incisions were made with a Thornton Triple Edged Arcuate diamond blade (Figure 14-6), available from Storz and Mastel. The blade extension was set for 100% of pachymetry reading at the 7mm optical zone, with the aim of achieving 98% depth in the incision.

As shown by topography, and confirmed by refraction, the coupling was markedly reduced, and at one week and three months post op his uncorrected vision was 20/25 and his refraction was -0.50 - 0.50 x 110 (Figure 14-7).

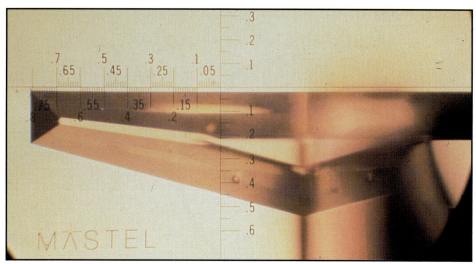

Figure 14-6. Thornton Triple Edged Arcuate Diamond Blade.

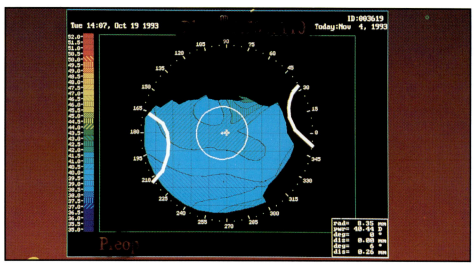

Figure 14-7. Topography confirms reduction of both cylinder and induced spherical myopia by inverse arcuate incisions.

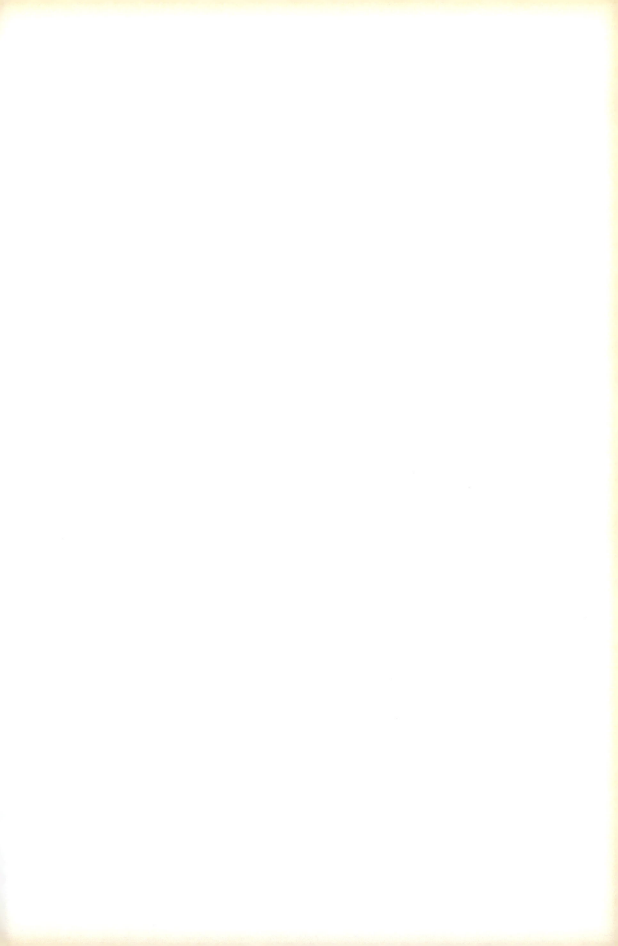

15

Complications of RK

Radial keratotomy has been shown to be a safe and effective procedure, but, as with any surgical procedure, complications can occur. Prevention of most complications is possible with precise preoperative planning, careful attention to intraoperative technique and careful adherence to a few rules.

Rules to Prevent Complications

1. Begin radial incisions at the optical zone.
2. Maintain stability of the eye with secure fixation.
3. Make all incisions slowly.
4. Don't incise the limbus.
5. Don't connect or cross incisions.
6. Set blade for precise depth under high power.
7. Mark visual axis and optical zone under high magnification.
8. Don't operate on a wet field.
9. Never irrigate an incision where microperforation has occurred.

Side Effects vs. Complications

A side effect is a difficulty frequently encountered, usually of limited nature, which does not alter the outcome. A complication is usually an unforeseen and unanticipated secondary condition which alters the course of treatment, making management difficult and the outcome uncertain.

A side effect, though it may cause difficulty for the patient, is the natural consequence of variable factors in the healing process and can, in most cases, be anticipated. Well known side effects of refractive surgery are fluctuation of vision, glare and photosensitivity, discomfort and tenderness and occasional diplopia.

The patient and physician should anticipate the known side effects by fully informing the patient prior to surgery. And, by carefully following the rules, most complications can be avoided.

Glare and Irregular Astigmatism

Glare and irregular astigmatism may be caused by inaccurate marking of the visual axis, using a too-small optical zone and invading the optical zone by one or more incisions.

The visual axis and the optical zone should be marked under high magnification to ensure proper centration. For most physicians this can be done binocularly. If the physician is not binocular a monocular method of marking the visual axis must be used (see Chapter 9, *Determining the Visual Axis*).

Binocular marking of the optical zone with low-profile markers under high magnification eliminates parallax problems and assures accurate optical zone margins. Invasion of the optical zone is avoided by beginning all radial incisions at the optical zone under precise control.

Technical Problems

Intraoperative complications can occur with all types of keratorefractive surgical procedures. Microperforations, inadvertent extension of incisions through the limbus, beveled or irregular incisions and too shallow incisions can all produce complications. Fortunately macroperforations and the possibility of anterior synechiae, hyphema, iritis and endophthalmitis are quite rare in the hands of experienced surgeons.

Incisions Into the Optical Zone

Incisions into the clear optical zone due to spontaneous eye movements and lack of surgical control is one of the most serious complications of the "uphill" or Russian-style technique. The most common cause of this problem is poor fixation and instability of the eye. Several methods of fixation have been used by refractive surgeons, each successful in varying degrees (depending on the skill of the surgeon) and each with its own proponents (Figure 15-1).

"Fixing on the light" is the *worst* type of fixation and amounts to no fixation at all in the opinion of a number of experienced refractive surgeons including this

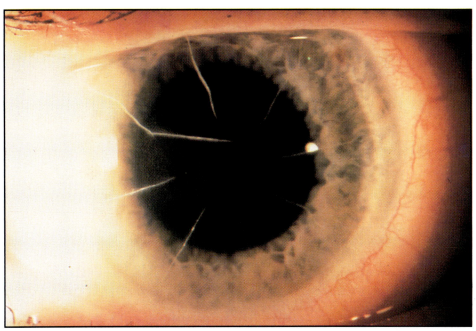

Figure 15-1. Invasion of the optical zone (OZ) by pushing the blade centrally with poor fixation.

author. Fixing on the light causes a shift of gaze when pressure is applied to the cornea and a decentering of the visual axis. This can be illustrated with pressure on your own eye while looking at a distant object. First, with both eyes open, press on the side of one eye through the upper eyelid. Diplopia is produced with the object of fixation shifting *toward* the point of pressure when pressure is applied close to the visual axis, and *away* from the point of pressure when pressure is applied peripherally.

When point pressure is applied to the eye with the fellow eye *closed*, a shift of the fixed object occurs *without* diplopia. When the patient is told to keep looking at the light, it should not be too surprising that an unexpected quick movement of the eye may occur as the surgeon pushes the blade toward the optical zone, with possibly disastrous results.

Forceps one or two point fixation can be effective in the hands of a highly skilled surgeon, but the weakness of one or two point fixation is that the intraocular pressure drops with every incision and the succeeding incisions tend to get shallower with lessening of effect in the area of the shallower incisions with induced astigmatism more likely (Figure 15-2).

Torque or lateral rotation of the eye is also more likely when fixation is inadequate, particularly when force vectors are directed toward the center of rotation as in the Russian method of cutting from the limbus toward the optical zone. On the other hand, if force vectors lead *away* from the center of rotation, torque does not occur.

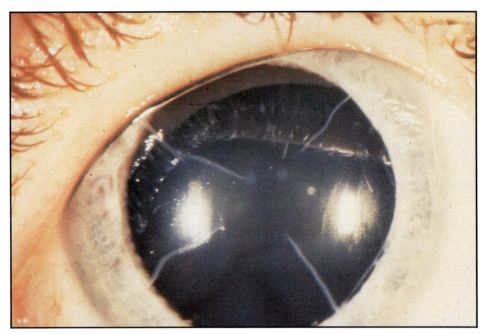

Figure 15-2. Pushing blade toward OZ produces torque with irregular incisions and invasion of OZ.

Most of the problems of fixation can be prevented by the secure fixation provided by a fixation ring. In addition, fixation with a fixation ring allows the surgeon to increase the intraocular pressure on the ring as each incision is made, helping to make the depth of the seventh or eighth incision the same as the first and second. Adequate fixation of the globe for absolute control of eye movement is a *must*, and ring fixation is the best method of achieving this.

Criticism of ring fixation is based on two things. First, the patient may feel the teeth of the ring. This problem is solved with adequate bulbar conjunctival topical anesthesia and properly manufactured fixation rings with short, non-sharp teeth. Second, there is the fear that as the ring is approached, the diamond blade may hit it and damage the diamond. This problem is solved by stopping before the ring is approached, lifting the diamond blade away from the eye, *moving* the ring, replacing it and continuing the incision.

By inserting the blade at the margin of the optical zone at the beginning of each incision it is virtually impossible to inadvertently incise the visual axis. And with the American system diamond blades now available, the tip and the back of the blade are easily seen as the blade is inserted at the edge of the optical zone. By *undercutting*, i.e., aiming the tip of the blade toward the center of the radius of curvature of the cornea (slightly anterior to the center of the globe) as it is inserted at the optical zone margin, the same "squared up" configuration of the incision at the optical zone margin is achieved with this American method as is claimed for the Russian technique. With firm fixation and precise control of the micrometer blade the incisions are consistently as deep and better controlled. This technique can be easily learned and mastered in wet-lab courses now being offered.

Perforations

Three things are important in preventing and managing perforations. One is accurate setting of the blade depth. Two is making all incisions slowly, and three, operating on a dry field so that the moment a microperforation is seen all motion can stop.

Accurate pachymetry performed in the office or in the operating room coupled with accurate extension of diamond blades prevent most microperforations, and by inserting the blade at the optical zone, waiting a few moments and then slowly moving the blade peripherally, macroperforations can be virtually eliminated.

By keeping the cornea dry any microperforation can be immediately detected, forward motion stopped and the knife withdrawn without any extension of the incision with resulting macroperforation.

The blade must be accurately set on the blade gauge under high magnification and double checked. Accurate pachymetry and precise measurement of blade extension prevents most perforations, but areas of undetected corneal thinning and excessive pressure on the blade may result in inadvertent perforation. The best way to avoid macroperforation is to operate on a dry field so that any microperforation is instantly seen. Microperforations self-seal very rapidly and early recognition will prevent extension into a macroperforation which requires suturing. The procedure does not have to be stopped.

If a microperforation occurs on the first incision, stop and recheck the extension of the blade under high magnification and, after allowing sufficient time for the perforation to seal, if the blade extension is accurate as determined preoperatively by pachymetry the second incision can be started 90° away. If no further perforations occur, complete all the incisions and come back to the perforated incision and insert the blade at the outer end of the incised area and with *light* pressure on the blade, move slowly toward the periphery to complete the incision. If any oozing is noted as the blade is inserted, *stop* and do not complete this incision.

If, on beginning the second incision (after one microperforation), a second microperforation is encountered, retract the blade 20 to 30mm and recheck your pachymetry readings before proceeding with further incisions. If no microperforation occurs on the second incision, all the other incisions can be completed and then return to the first incision, retract the blade 20mm and continue from the point of microperforation toward the periphery with a "light touch."

If your pachymetry has shown an area of corneal thinning, leave that area until last and when you get to that area move very *slowly* with *light pressure*. Though the inferior temporal cornea tends to be thinnest, areas of thinning can occur anywhere in the cornea, pointing out the importance of preoperative pachymetry of the entire cornea. If a microperforation occurs on incision number three or four you have greater assurance that you have encountered an area of unforeseen thinning or minimal over extension of the blade which can be managed by retracting the blade 20mm before continuing.

To retract a diamond blade 20mm you should first retract 100mm using the micrometer handle, then advance 80mm. Micrometer extension is more accurate than micrometer retraction.

If the perforation is macro rather than micro and continues to leak, a single 11-0 nylon or 11-0 mersilene suture will seal the opening and the suture can be removed within two weeks.

Another technique of avoiding perforations on subsequent incisions is to avoid putting undue pressure on the cornea with the blade or on the globe with the fixation ring.

Extension of Incisions Into the Limbus

Another intraoperative complication which can produce variable results is extending the incisions beyond the clear cornea into or beyond the limbus. Possible vascularization of the incision tracks along with destabilization of the cornea with subsequent progression of effect may result. This can be avoided by carrying the incisions through the limbal arcade but stopping short of the corneal-scleral junction.

Intersection of Incisions

Intersection of incisions occurs more readily when the incisions are pushed from the periphery to the optical zone and when larger numbers of incisions are used. The maximum number of radial incisions in any one procedure should be limited to eight. The intersection of incisions is a complication that should be avoided as corneal gape inevitably results with poor wound healing and resulting irregular astigmatism (Figure 15-3). If incision intersection occurs, the surgeon should use 11 - 0 nylon or mersilene sutures to reapproximate the gaped margins. The knots should be buried and the sutures left in place for 3-4 months. Failure to repair the wound gape results in collagen and epithelial ingrowth with wound destabilization.

In cases in which healing has occurred with epithelial ingrowth, the treatment consists of opening the incisions and scraping the epithelium from the incisions with a micro-spatula and reapproximating the edges with 11-0 mersilene or nylon with the knots buried. The sutures should remain in place for 4 - 6 months.

Recurrent Corneal Erosions

Recurrent erosions and stromal disorders can occur if incisions are crossed (Figure 15-4). In addition, several conditions may predispose to recurrent erosion and stromal melt. If the patient's history reveals a history of severe dry eye or keratitis sicca or systemic autoimmune disorders, incisional keratotomy is contraindicated. In patients with significantly diminished tear production, punctal occlusion should be considered before incisional keratotomy is considered.

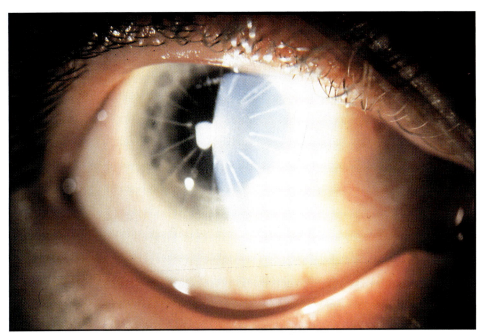

Figure 15-3. Intersecting incisions result in poor wound healing.

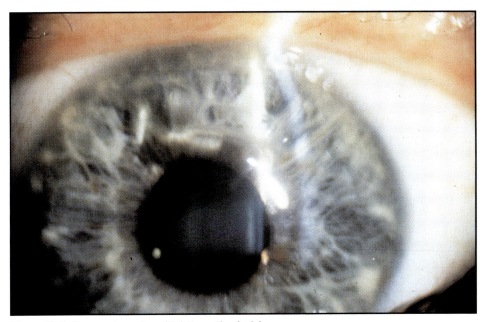

Figure 15-4. Recurrent erosion with intersecting incisions.

Induced Irregular Astigmatism

The most common clinical finding with irregular astigmatism is decreased best-corrected visual acuity. This can occur with any keratorefractive procedure in which the optical zone is irregularly placed or if incisions are placed asymmetrically around the visual axis. When this is detected or suspected the eye should be examined frequently and treated conservatively. No additional incisions should be placed to correct the astigmatism until the refraction and topography have completely stabilized.

Over Aggressive Management

Especially in astigmatic keratotomy it is a commonly made mistake to perform additional surgery before the eye has had a chance to stabilize. Allowing a several month interval between surgical procedures will frequently show that further surgery is not actually necessary.

Corneal topography is indispensable in determining the extent and location of persistent irregular astigmatism and tracking its change over time. Intervening too soon with corrective procedures may make the situation worse and the astigmatism ultimately more difficult to correct. Conservative management with repeated corneal topography over a period of time can help determine whether subsequent incisions are necessary, and their optimal location.

Undercorrection and Overcorrection

By careful preoperative planning and following the nomogram precisely, you can come very close to the targeted result in all but a few cases in which unforeseen biological variables produce variation. The surgeon should always aim at a slight undercorrection of myopia to avoid even minimal overcorrection. If the undercorrection is great enough to cause problems you can always do an "enhancement" but it is good to remember that there is no eraser on the end of the blade and overcorrections and progression of effect are best treated by avoiding them whenever possible by a conservative approach to the initial procedure.

The most effective treatment of overcorrection is to reopen the incisions and scrape out any epithelial inclusions or fibrovascular tracks and reapproximating the incision margins with interrupted 10-0 mersilene sutures at the 6 or 7mm optical zone. The sutures should be about 75% deep, relatively tight and extend about 1/2mm to either side of the incision. They should be left in place indefinitely, and be removed only if necessary.

Significant unplanned undercorrections may be further corrected by enhancement, "fine tuning" or re-operation. The patient should have been prepared for this possibility pre-operatively by explaining "staging" of surgery to attain the most desirable level of vision without overcorrection.

If significant undercorrection is apparent at the first or second week examination and you do not get a prompt and satisfactory steroid response, enhancement or re-operation should be considered.

To determine whether to recut the original incisions to get deeper cuts and a smaller optical zone, examine the eye carefully under the slit lamp microscope and: a) if the incisions appear shallow, deepen the original incisions; b) if the incisions are short or not deep at the optical zone, lengthen the incisions at the optical zone, cutting deep at the optical zone, and; c) if the incisions appear deep and at the proper optical zone, add new incisions. If a or b is the case, do enhancement as soon as possible. If c is the case, wait at least six to eight weeks for additional incisions to allow stabilization of the refraction.

Progression of Effect

A gradual post-operative hyperopic shift or progression of effect of the radial keratotomy may be related to smaller optical zones, number of incisions, crossing the limbus, rubbing the eyes and/or failure to account for latent hyperopia by not doing cycloplegic refraction at the time of pre-operative evaluation. Thus progressive hyperopia may be due to a combination of factors.

Idiopathic: Elevated intraocular pressure and unforeseen biological factors such as latent hyperopia.

Iatrogenic: Small optical zones and greater number of incisions, crossing the limbus and cutting the peripheral circular ligament.

Patient Induced: Rubbing the eyes.

The most likely cause of progressive hyperopia, however, is incising too deeply in the extreme periphery of the cornea in the area of the ligamentum circulare (the "ligament of Kokutt") with loss of the restraining strength of the circumferential "belt" of the cornea. Without this belt the cornea can continue to expand with any internal pressure over the years, and with stimuli such as increased IOP, rubbing the eye, external pressures on the eye during sleep, etc. the inevitable result is increased stretch on the central cornea and increased flattening centrally.

I recommend deepening of incisions from optical zones well away from the extreme periphery and, except in cases where I want to get the absolute maximum effect, I deepen from the 5 or the 7mm optical zones. In cases where I have more than 7 diopters myopia to correct I use 8 incisions redeepened at the 5 and the 7mm optical zone with the blade fully extended to get an *achieved* depth of 98% in the area of the 5 and 7mm optical zone.

Incision Abnormalities

Epithelial ingrowth and transient epithelial disruptions may result from cellular inclusions at the time of surgery, emphasizing the desirability of irrigation of incisions at the conclusion of the procedure. Collagenous adhesion within the incision may require up to six weeks or longer to mature and anything trapped within the incision tracks may delay the process. Foreign material, including mascara, epithelial inclusion cysts, blood cells, powder from the surgical gloves, and crystals from eye drop suspensions may become trapped within the incision tracks. Most of this material extrudes over a period of two or three months without sequelae but careful saline irrigation of the incisions at the conclusion of surgery is the best treatment.

Anesthetic Complications and Optic Nerve Damage

Optic nerve damage is completely avoidable. Experience has taught us that local anesthesia with peribulbar or retrobulbar injection is completely unnecessary with radial keratotomy and astigmatic keratotomy. Deep topical anesthesia has been shown to be completely effective in eliminating pain and discomfort with instrumentation related to radial keratotomy and astigmatic keratotomy.

Prior to surgery the eye is anesthetized by first retracting the lower lid and dropping one drop of Proparicaine (ophthaine) in the lower cul-de-sac. After a few seconds the upper lid is retracted and the second drop instilled in the upper cul-de-sac. Wait fifteen to twenty seconds and retract the lower lid and place another drop in the cul-de-sac and after another few seconds retract the upper lid again and place another drop in the upper cul-de-sac. This process is repeated six or eight times over a period of two or three minutes. Just prior to marking the optical zone and prior to any incisions the anesthetic effect is enhanced with 4% Xylocaine (lidocaine) drops to produce a topical anesthetic effect which lasts for several hours.

Greater comfort for the patient and easier stabilization of the eye and avoidance of any possible optic nerve damage or retrobulbar hemorrhage is the advantage of topical anesthesia.

Infection

The most serious sight threatening complication associated with refractive surgery is infectious keratitis, and may occur in close proximity to surgery in the post operative period, or may be associated with later contact lens wear.

The risk of infection is best anticipated by examining patients for blepharitis preoperatively and prophylactically prescribing broad spectrum antibiotic eye drops before and after surgery.

Sterile technique should be observed during refractive surgery with the use of sterile gloves and masks by personnel within the operating area. The surgical field should be prepped with Betadine and the same precautions observed as in cataract surgery.

Patients should be warned against rubbing the eyes and should be instructed to avoid eye makeup and exposure to swimming pools and hot tubs for one week after surgery.

Early detection of infection is critical. The patient should be instructed to call with any unusual pain or redness and should be examined the day following surgery and within one week after.

If infiltrates are detected in the deep stroma they must be presumed to be bacterial and the epithelium over the incision in the involved area should be opened, and stains and cultures obtained from the inside of the incision. Intensive broad spectrum antibiotic therapy should be started immediately while waiting for culture results.

Ancef, Tobramycin and Norfloxacin may be effective when given in rotation every 30 minutes. A combination of 0.4cc Ancef and 0.4cc Tobramycin mixed with 0.1cc of 2% lidocaine hydrochloride can be administered as a subconjunctival injection in the affected area daily until culture results are available or there is significant clinical improvement. The overlying epithelium should be debrided to enable high concentrations of antibiotic penetration to the deep stroma. Steroids should never be used with deep stromal keratitis.

With early detection and prompt treatment most complications can be successfully treated.

Summary

Despite the outstanding results achieved by refractive surgery, a variety of complications have been reported, and complications such as overreactions, corneal erosions, recurrent keratitis, progressive hyperopia and induced astigmatism can and do occur and other complications will probably be reported.

A side effect, though it may cause difficulty for the patient, is the natural consequence of variable factors in the healing process and can, in most cases, be anticipated. Well known side effects of refractive surgery are fluctuation of vision, glare and photosensitivity, discomfort and tenderness and occasional diplopia.

Intraoperative complications can occur with all types of keratorefractive surgical procedures. Microperforations, inadvertent extension of incisions through limbal vessels, beveled or irregular incisions and too-shallow incisions can all produce complications. Fortunately, macroperforations and the possibility of anterior synechiae, hyphema, iritis and endophthalmitis are quite rare in the hands of experienced surgeons.

Inadequate Preparation

Inadequate preparation may result in incisions in the wrong meridian or off axis, producing unwanted and unexpected refractive errors. Astigmatic procedures performed off axis will produce a shift of the astigmatic error making further correction even more difficult. Operating on the wrong meridian or choosing the wrong procedure for a specific error can produce unwanted results. For example, a modified Ruiz procedure on an eye whose spherical equivalent is plano will correct the astigmatism but will increase the patient's hyperopia.

Optical Zone Errors

Performing radial keratotomy with an optical zone smaller than 3mm is risking the possibility of severe glare problems, and the risk of slight displacement of the optical zone becomes increasingly greater with smaller optical zones—therefore a minimum limit of 3mm is recommended. In astigmatic keratotomy an optical zone smaller than 5mm not only increases the probability of glare problems but increases the chance of induced irregular astigmatism and other optical errors. I personally prefer using a 6mm optical zone as the minimum for transverse incisions.

Non-inflammatory complications of refractive surgery should be treated cautiously and conservatively. Many things are labeled complications which, with time, are shown to be variations in the healing process.

16

Re-operations

Enhancements

Enhancements or "fine tuning" and "re-ops" are euphemistic ways of describing secondary surgery in cases where a satisfactory level of vision was not achieved with the first procedure. Because of unpredictable biological variables and variations in intraoperative approach, secondary procedures are occasionally necessary and should be anticipated at the time of the initial patient evaluation and explanation of surgery. The patient should be informed that "staging" of surgery may be necessary to attain the most desirable level of vision, but every attempt will be made to obtain maximal correction with the first procedure.

It is important to learn how to present the possibility of enhancement surgery to your patients so that both you and your patient are comfortable. It is helpful to have guidelines in deciding who to enhance and how to enhance properly in order to maximize your success rate with secondary procedures.

Though it is our objective to correct as much of the myopic and astigmatic error as possible in the first procedure, patients tend to accept the conservative attitude that, "it is better to slightly under-correct than over-correct" and fine tuning with enhancements may be necessary in the process of bringing them to 20/40 or better uncorrected. It is easier to increase the effect of under-correction with fine tuning than to reverse the effect of an over-response.

A positive attitude by you and your staff in the post-operative period after the primary procedure is critical. Your staff should not relay to the patient the residual refractive error in numbers. The nurse or technician can help maintain a positive attitude by emphasizing the pre-operative uncorrected visual acuity and what a positive difference has been made with the improved post-operative visual acuity without correction.

In planning enhancements it is better to be guided by the patient's comments regarding his or her needs than to be guided strictly by acuity. If the patient is satisfied, *do not enhance.* Many times the uncorrected acuity is better than expected for the amount of measured residual error in post-op RK patients because of the larger retinal image produced by the changed corneal curvature.

A presbyopic patient with uncorrected 20/25 vision in one eye and 20/50 in the other with residual myopia may be quite content because he or she can see well at distance and read without glasses. When this type of patient insists on enhancement surgery to get "both eyes perfect at distance," I put their distance correction in trial frames and demonstrate to them the amount of reading ability they will be giving up because of their presbyopia. Most then realize the benefits of this slight undercorrection and decide that they are happy with the result after all.

System Differences

The systems which promote limbus to optical zone cuts claim that their cuts are deeper and more precise. And yet it is those very systems which admit to having to enhance up to 40% of their cases one or two or *more* times before they are adequately corrected and their emphasis is on "making their *original incisions* adequately deep." Apparently these systems are not as precise or as reproducible as they have led themselves to believe. Precision requires thought and attention to detail. It cannot be achieved by "cookbook" technology.

Enhancements should *not* be an integral part of state-of-the-art refractive surgery! Any system of surgery that leads to a high percentage of re-operations should be viewed with caution. To advocate re-operations or enhancements as part of the original surgical plan is to admit that the approach advocated is trial and error.

The American system that I've used and taught since 1981, with its known modifiers and time-proven nomograms, is designed to reduce the need for enhancements. Overcorrections are unlikely with this system's nomograms, as several safety factors are built-in. But enhancements *are* necessary in a few cases and the patient must be prepared *before surgery* for the possibility of the patient under-responding or over-responding to surgery.

Indications for Enhancement

Significant undercorrection after radial keratotomy is probably present when the patient states that vision is good in the morning but gets blurry or out of focus in the afternoon or evening. On the other hand, if the vision is blurry in the morning and clears up in the afternoon, *overcorrection* is likely.

If the post-op best corrected vision is less than pre-op, irregular astigmatism is likely. Irregular astigmatism may be manifested by monocular diplopia, halos and decreased corrected acuity both for near and distance. A number of studies have shown that repeated enhancements are more likely to cause irregular astigmatism than carefully done primary procedures. Therefore the fewer procedures done the better.

Determining the Need for Enhancement

When undercorrection is demonstrated by patient complaint and confirmed by morning and afternoon refraction, enhancement may be necessary. If, within the first week or so, the surgeon can diagnose at the slit lamp the cause of the under-correction, such as short or shallow incisions, an early enhancement is called for. It is relatively easy to enhance at this stage because the incisions open easily with a Sinskey hook and a Thornton incision spreader and they can be opened so that the square tipped Triple Edged Arcuate diamond blade can be accurately inserted in the original incisions at the newly measured pachymetry depth.

Re-Cut Original Incisions Or Add New Incisions

To determine whether to re-cut the original incisions to get deeper cuts or a smaller optical zone, examine the eye carefully under the slit lamp microscope and: a) if the incisions appear shallow, deepen the original incisions; b) if the incisions are short or not deep at the optical zone, lengthen the incisions at the optical zone, cutting deep at the optical zone line; c) if the incisions appear deep and at the proper optical zone, add new incisions.

When Should Enhancements Be Done?

If undercorrection is apparent at the first or second week examination (if a or b above is the case) and you do not get a prompt and satisfactory steroid response, plan enhancement surgery as soon as possible.

If c is the case and there is no clear evidence of shallow or short incisions, it is best to wait at least two or three months before adding additional incisions to allow stabilization of the refraction. Apparent undercorrections may be caused by sub-clinical stromal edema and may spontaneously improve with time. A good rule of thumb is to wait as long as possible before proceeding with repeat surgery, because if you overcorrect with your enhancement it is most difficult to undo it.

The Surgical Approach to Enhancements

One should look at the uncorrected visual acuity, the residual refractive error and best corrected visual acuity, the computer assisted corneal topography analysis, and the incision profile. The incision profile is the appearance of the ends of the incision at the central optical zone and at the periphery. A more "squared off" profile provides more flattening effect than a "sloping" profile.

The incision depth is determined by viewing the incision under the slit lamp under high power and determining how much the incision occupies the depth of the illuminated corneal "slice of light." Another method of evaluation is to determine how much unincised tissue fills the posterior portion of the slit beam. An estimate of depth in that area is then determined. Remember that the actual depth may be a little deeper with the newer, thinner diamond blades.

Obtainable Effect With More Surgery

A number of studies have shown that with eight-incision radial keratotomy the first four incisions correct about 65% of the total. Therefore if you have done a four-incision case and the result is 35 - 40% less than desired, you can do another four incisions at or near the same optical zone for the desired total effect.

Relative Effect of RK Incisions	
Incision #	% of Total Effect
1	20 - 25%
2	35 - 40%
3	50 - 55%
4	60 - 65%
5	70 - 75%
6	80 - 85%
7	90 - 95%
8	100%

With Small Undercorrections

In four-incision cases, if the remaining error is under 25% of the original target error and there is room for deepening, you may obtain satisfactory correction of the remainder by deepening the original incisions to the original optical zone.

If the undercorrection is 25% or less than the desired target amount and you would rather add four more incisions, you can use a larger optical zone for additional incisions than in the original procedure in your re-operation, but *only* if the undercorrection is 25% or less.

When undercorrection occurs with an optical zone of 3.5mm or more and re-operation is desired, the amount of remaining error determines the type of secondary procedure to be planned.

For Moderate Undercorrections

If the remaining error is 30 to 35% of the original intended correction you may get satisfactory correction by adding four more incisions at the *same* optical zone at maximal depth. If you use the same optical zone as in the original procedure you can achieve the level of correction that would have been achieved if eight incisions had been done originally. If the remaining error is more than 40% of the original error you will need to bring your additional incisions to a *smaller* optical zone. Since shallow incisions may be part of the cause of the undercorrection you must be *sure* that any added incisions are of *maximal depth* (even at the risk of getting a microperforation).

The optical zone must be rechecked and re-marked and pachymetry rechecked at the point of entry for any new or extended incisions.

Recalculate the amount of correction desired and tailor the re-operation procedure to the specific case. Remember that you are no longer operating on a "virgin" cornea and additional incisions do not give the same effect as the original ones.

Never be too quick to attempt correction of astigmatic undercorrection or apparent axis shift. Stabilization of the cornea may take several months and you may end up "chasing" the astigmatism around the cornea by being too aggressive. Reassure the patient that the eye is gradually adapting to its changed circumference (remember that all incisions act as if tissue is added and post operative edema may mimic under or over-correction at least temporarily) and with stabilization may come visual improvement.

Don't be too ready to enhance. If you are at all unsure, give the patient the option of temporary spectacles. It is important not to enhance for the wrong reasons. Allowing an adequate time interval between surgical procedures frequently shows that further surgery is not actually necessary. If the patient wants enhancement because of glare and fluctuating vision, another procedure may worsen their symptoms. A temporary spectacle lens will allow time for the symptoms to resolve and give time for the refractive error to stabilize. Demonstrating to the patient that he is correctable to his best pre-op vision with "much less correction" is reassuring and frequently results in a happy patient without having to re-operate.

Improving Your Success Rate

The variables that lead to less than satisfactory results are for the most part identifiable and correctable. The equipment, instrumentation, and the nomograms are integrated into a unified whole which is referred to as a "system." And yes, this means that the instruments used in one system may not produce the desired results with another system's technique. The most important part of any system however, is the surgeon.

Taking short-cuts and maintaining a casual attitude are frequently associated with a higher enhancement rate, with the surgeon thinking, "If I don't get it right the first time, I can always re-do it."

Repeat surgery is frequently necessary because of errors in surgical planning. Calculation errors may result in either overcorrection or undercorrection. These errors may be from any of several sources.

Sources of Error

Errors may result if the wrong information is used to derive the theoretical error, for example the wrong age, the wrong corneal thickness, wrong keratometry, or by using the spherical component in plus cylinder form or using the spherical equivalent when the cylinder is not being corrected.

Errors may result when the wrong refraction is used. The plus cylinder is used rather than the minus, or the spherical equivalent was calculated *after* applying modifiers (improper conversion to spherical equivalent).

Errors can occur when the pachymetry is not done in each area of the cornea where incisions are to be made, or when there is an instrument malfunction or when the instrument is misread.

Errors can occur when the wrong axis is determined for the astigmatism (remember, the *plus* cylinder tells you the axis of the cornea which is steep, across which transverse incisions should be placed, and the *minus* cylinder tells you the proper amount of myopia for correction). *Never* use the spherical equivalent to correct the myopia unless you are going to correct the cylinder.

Technical Considerations

Errors may occur with an incorrect optical zone. This may occur in referring to the nomogram, but more commonly it occurs when the surgeon stops short of the planned optical zone, or when he violates the optical zone by pushing the blade into it (with the Russian system). This is avoided by using the American system approach and inserting the tip of the blade precisely into the edge of the optical zone at the beginning of each incision.

Errors can occur when the incisions are too shallow or when the blade extension is improperly set, particularly when incorrect corneal depth is calculated (especially when only one pachymetry reading is done), when the corneal surface is not fully applanated by the micrometer footplates (not uncommon when there is poor fixation of the eye) or when the blade is tilted sideways or angled forward or backward.

In many cases the surgeon can identify the cause of error and correct it, by proper equipment (pachymeter, diamond blades, proper markers, gauges, etc.), accurate application of the nomogram, proper setting of the blade, correct optical zone, etc., and markedly reduce the number of enhancements needed.

You should attempt to correct as much of the myopic and astigmatic error as possible in the first operation and leave the enhancements or "re-ops" to those cases where biological and technical variables have led to significant undercorrection.

17

Management of Overcorrection

Overcorrection may be seen following any surgical procedure designed to correct refractive errors. If seen following radial keratotomy or astigmatic keratotomy for myopia or myopic astigmatism, I recommend the following steps:

1. Immediately *stop* steroids.

2. Immediately begin Pilocarpine 1/2% q.i.d.

3. Immediately begin Timoptic or other topical beta-blocker b.i.d.

4. Start on Diamox unless allergic to sulfas.

5. Immediately start Muro 128 (hypertonic saline) drops at least q.i.d. and Muro 128 Ointment at bedtime daily.

6. Start frequent lubricant eye drops (AquaSite, Hypotears, etc.).

7. Strongly caution against rubbing the eye.

8. Be patient! Though improvement may be noted within the first few weeks, several months of treatment may be required for stability.

Surgical Treatment of Overcorrection

Numerous methods of correcting overcorrections have been reported, but none have received wide acceptance. The approaches reported have included "purse-string" sutures placed circumferentially at the 5, 6 or 7mm optical zone, interrupted sutures placed across the radials at any of several optical zones, and procedures such as hexagonal keratotomy, thermal keratoplasty, and lamellar keratectomy. At the time of this writing, no one method has been shown to be markedly superior or universally applicable.

Suturing Radials

With overcorrections up to 3.0 diopters I have found the following technique to be useful. Under topical anesthesia, and centered on the visual axis, mark the cornea with a 7.0mm optical zone marker stained with gentian violet. If transverse incisions are present in the 7.0mm optical zone then use a 6.0mm zone marker.

Open each incision with a Sinskey hook by pressing the hook into the incision near the limbus. When it is open a millimeter or so, insert the tip of the Thornton Incision Spreader (Storz) into the opening and open the incision up to the optical zone. Run the blades of the incision spreader back and forth in the incision to "debride" the edges with the sand-blasted sides of the incision spreader. Then irrigate the incision with BSS on an irrigating canula.

Place a 10-0 Mersilene or Prolene suture across the incision at the 7.0mm mark. Take a good, deep bite about 1mm to each side of the incision and tie the suture with compression. Although each suture may open up the adjacent incision, you will be placing a suture across each incision by the time you finish.

With overcorrections over 3.0 diopters, place *two* sutures across each incision, one at the 6.0mm zone and one at the 8.0mm zone. Tie each with compression and pull the knots below the surface.

The tight sutures will steepen the central cornea, just as a tight suture at the limbus will steepen the cornea. The cornea is allowed to heal in this splinted condition for several months. The immediate effect will be to make the patient myopic, and most of the time will also induce some astigmatism due to irregularity in tension on the sutures. This irregularity will decrease over the first two or three months as the tightest sutures loosen a bit.

Following the progress of healing with periodic topography will allow you to monitor the changes in the astigmatism and allow you to titrate the effect with selective removal of sutures as necessary after the first three or four months. I think that three or four months is adequate for keeping the sutures in place. But if the resulting correction is good and the patient is not bothered by any surface irregularity, I would leave the sutures in indefinitely.

In the post operative period the eye should be treated by antibiotic drops q.i.d. for the first few weeks, but do not use any topical steroids, since you are trying to promote rapid healing. The patient also must be repeatedly cautioned not to rub the eye, lie with the eye on the arm, etc. IOP lowering measures should also be carried out during the healing period to prevent any loosening of the sutures.

18

Current and Future Trends

Ophthalmology has experienced tremendous changes over the last two decades, with the acceptance and increasing popularity of intraocular lenses and more recently with the recognition of refractive surgery as a natural consequence of recent advances in cataract and IOL surgery.

Radial and astigmatic keratotomy are finding their way into the repertoire of an increasing number of cataract surgeons because cataract surgery itself is now recognized as a refractive procedure. With smaller incisions and foldable, injectable intraocular lenses, the correction of both spherical and cylindrical errors are within the reach of the average cataract surgeon.

Toric IOLs have been shown to be effective in the correction of low degrees of astigmatism, and the combination of incision placement, incision architecture and concurrent relaxing corneal incisions have been shown effective in correcting larger degrees of pre-existing astigmatism.

The Mission of Refractive Surgery

In addition to the restoration of sight in cataract patients, the aim of the progressive ophthalmologist is to provide a means of improved quality of life, and refractive surgery has been shown to be effective in meeting that need. The high level of patient satisfaction and gratitude make for a specialty that provides much more than monetary reward. A variety of procedures are developing to improve the odds of providing emmetropia to individuals with all types of visual problems, not just myopia.

From lasers to lamellar keratoplasty to intraocular contact lenses, the field of corrective visual surgery is positioned for certain growth in the future. The options open to the ophthalmologist are increasing as laser technology improves and comes on-line. But will the laser completely supplant incisional refractive surgery? I don't think so.

The Future of RK

Radial keratotomy has been shown to be most effective and most predictable in lower ranges, up to about six or seven diopters. Above that range the predictability decreases and multiple procedures (enhancements) become more common. Both lamellar keratoplasty and laser surgery have been shown to be effective in higher degrees of error. In addition, the potential for correcting hyperopic errors with either lamellar keratoplasty or laser procedures make these approaches desirable over incisional surgery in this type error.

It appears then, that laser surgery and RK will be mutually complementary and will co-exist in the armamentarium of the progressive ophthalmologist in his or her quest for the safest and most effective methods of producing emmetropia in myopic, astigmatic and cataract patients.

Appendix A

Thornton Nomograms

Thornton Nomogram For Radial Keratotomy

Requisites: Centrifugal incisions, cycloplegic refraction, 90% achieved *average* depth (98% at optical zone) and redeepening of all radial incisions for increased effect when indicated (see below).

Factors considered: Refractive Error, Age, Sex, Intraocular Pressure, Corneal Thickness, Corneal Diameter and Keratometry.
The Sum of all these Factors = the Working Sphere (Theoretical)

Age: For every year below age 30 add 2% to the myopic error. For every year above age 30 subtract 2% from the myopic error to age 50, then 1% per year thereafter to age 75.

Sex: Subtract 3 years from age for premenopausal females to age 40.

IOP: For every mm IOP below 12 add 2% to the myopic refractive error. For every mm IOP above 15, subtract 2% from the myopic refractive error.

Corneal Thickness: For central corneal thickness less than 490μ, add 10% to the myopia. From 490 to 510, add 5%. From 510 to 580 make no change. From 580 to 600 subtract 5%, and above 600 subtract 10% from the myopia.

Corneal Diameter: If the corneal diameter is less than 11.5mm, add 10% to the myopic error. If the corneal diameter is greater than 12.5mm, subtract 10% from the myopic error.

Keratometry: If the average K is 42.75 or less, add 10% to the myopia. From 42.75 to 43.50, add 5%. From 43.50 to 46.00, make no change. From 46.00 to 46.75, subtract 5%. If the average K is 46.75 or more, subtract 10% from the myopia.

Advanced Radial Keratotomy Technique: Titration of Effect

Four incisions would be expected to give results in the lower half of any given range and eight would be expected to give results in the upper half. Back-cutting or "squaring up" from the limbus will assure the maximum correction possible with a single pass in any given optical zone. Redeepening increases the effect from 0.50 to 0.75D with either four or eight incisions. Deepening all incisions to 98% from the 7mm optical zone adds approximately 0.50D to the correction and deepening to 98% from the 5mm optical zone adds approximately 0.75D to the correction.

Thornton Nomogram for Radial Keratotomy (continued)

Theoretical Working Sphere Range of Myopic Power	Optical Zone (Number of Incisions in parentheses)
0.75 — 1.12	5.00 (8) 4.75 (4)
1.13 — 1.49	4.75 (8) 4.50 (4)
1.50 — 2.11	4.50 (8) 4.25 (4)
2.12 — 2.61	4.25 (8) 4.00 (4)
2.62 — 3.11	4.00 (8) 3.75 (4)
3.12 — 3.73	3.75 (8) 3.50 (4)
3.75 — 4.36	3.50 (8) 3.25 (4)
4.37 — 5.11	3.25 (8) 3.00 (4)
5.12 — 6.11	3.00 (8)
6.12 — 7.50	3.00 (8 & redeepen to 98% from 5mm OZ)
7.51 — 8.00 or more	3.00 (8 & redeepen to 98% from 5 and 7mm OZ)

Thornton Nomogram for Astigmatic Keratotomy

Assumes cuts 98% deep (almost to Decemet's Membrane) along the full length of the incision.

Age: For every year below age 30 add 1/2% to the astigmatic error. For every year above age 30 subtract 1/2%.

Sex: In premenopausal women (under age 40) subtract three years from actual age.

IOP: For every mm IOP below 12 add 2% to the astigmatic error. For every mm IOP above 15, subtract 2%.

Add or subtract the sum of the modifiers (%)
from the actual amount of cylinder for the "Theoretical Cylinder."

Cylinder Corrected by Paired Arcuate Transverse Incisions

Chord Length of One Pair
Arcuate Transverse Incisions

Theoretical Cylinder	Degrees Arc
0.50 D	20°
0.75 D	23°
1.00 D	25°
1.25 D	28°
1.50 D	32°
1.75 D	35°
2.00 D	38°
2.25 D	42°
2.50 D	45°

One pair
always placed at
the 7 mm OZ

Thornton Nomogram for Astigmatic Keratotomy (continued)

Chord Length of Two Pairs
Arcuate Transverse Incisions

Theoretical Cylinder	Degrees Arc
2.00 D	23°
2.25 D	27°
2.50 D	31°
2.75 D	35°
3.00 D	39°
3.25 D	43°
3.50 D	47°
3.75 D	50°

Two pairs
outer at the 8
inner at the 6

Chord Length of Three Pairs
Arcuate Transverse Incisions

Theoretical Cylinder	Degrees Arc
3.25 D	22°
3.50 D	26°
3.75 D	30°
4.00 D	35°
4.25 D	40°
4.50 D	45°
4.75 D	50°
5.00 D	54°

Three pairs
outer just outside the 8
middle incision at the 7
inner just inside the 6

Smaller OZ (5.5 mm to 7.5 mm) -0.50 D to 1.00 D more

Thornton Nomogram for Astigmatic Keratotomy with Inverse Arcuate Incisions

Assumes cuts 98% deep (almost to Descemet's Membrane) along the full length of the incision.

Age: For every year below 30 add 1/2% to the astigmatic error. For every year above age 30 subtract 1/2%.

Sex: In pre-menopausal women (under age 40) subtract three years from actual age.

IOP: For every mm IOP below 12 add 2% to the astigmatic error. For every mm IOP above 15, subtract 2%.

Add or subtract the sum of the modifiers (%) from the actual amount of cylinder for the "Theoretical Cylinder."

Inverse arc incisions, because of their transverse *and* radial components, *cancel out any potential coupling* but retain their meridional flattening potential because their arc length is based on established concentric arcuate incision lengths (the Thornton Astigmatic Keratotomy Nomograms).

The optical zones given are for the *mid-point* of the inverse arc. Single pairs of incisions are always placed mid-point at the 7mm optical zone. Double pairs of incisions are always placed mid-point on the 6 and 7mm optical zone, and three pairs are always placed with the mid-point of the inner pair just inside the 6mm optical zone, the middle pair placed mid-point on the 7mm optical zone and the third, outer, pair placed mid-point just touching outside the 8mm OZ.

Thornton Nomogram for Astigmatic Keratotomy with Inverse Arcuate Incisions (continued)

Cylinder Corrected by Paired Inverse Arcuate Incisions

Chord Length of One Pair Inverse Arcuate Incisions

Theoretical Cylinder	Degrees Arc
1.00 D	25°
1.25 D	28°
1.50 D	32°
1.75 D	35°
2.00 D	38°
2.25 D	42°
2.50 D	45°

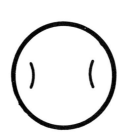 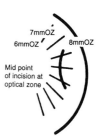

Chord Length of Two Pairs Inverse Arcuate Incisions

Theoretical Cylinder	Degrees Arc
2.00 D	23°
2.25 D	27°
2.50 D	31°
2.75 D	35°
3.00 D	39°
3.25 D	43°
3.50 D	47°
3.75 D	50°

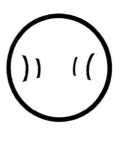 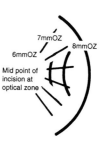

Chord Length of Three Pairs Inverse Arcuate Incisions

Theoretical Cylinder	Degrees Arc
3.25 D	22°
3.50 D	26°
3.75 D	30°
4.00 D	35°
4.25 D	40°
4.50 D	45°
4.75 D	50°
5.00 D	54°

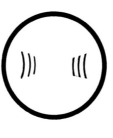 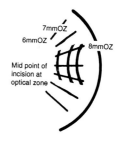

Appendix B

Centering Corneal Surgical Procedures

Hiroshi Uozato, PhD., and David L. Guyton, MD

ABSTRACT

Currently used methods for centering corneal surgical procedures emphasize the visual axis of the eye but do not define it properly. We obtained the best optical result by centering the surgical procedure on the line of sight and entrance pupil of the eye, not on the visual axis. We found an error of 0.5 to 0.8mm in currently used methods of marking the visual axis, which arose from the use of the corneal light reflex as a sighting point or from inadvertent monocular sighting in techniques requiring binocular sighting. Proper centering requires the patient to fixate on a point that is coaxial with the surgeon's sighting eye, and the cornea is marked at the point in line with the center of the patient's entrance pupil, ignoring the corneal light reflex.

We believe that even if the true visual axis could be located, it is the center of the entrance pupil, not the visual axis, that should be used for centering corneal surgical procedures.

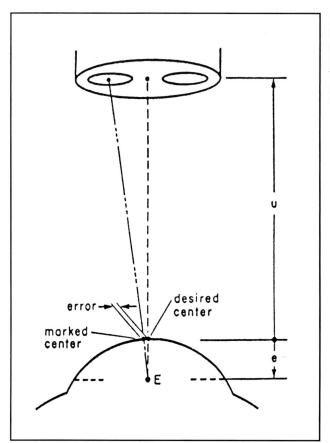

Figure 1. (Uozato and Guyton). Schematic illustration of the error in corneal centering caused by monocular sighting of the center of the pupil as the patient fixates Thornton's nonluminous fixation target.

Entrance Pupil and Line of Sight

When we look at an eye, we do not actually see the real pupil and iris; we see a virtual image of the pupil and iris formed by the cornea. The virtual image of the pupil is called the entrance pupil of the eye. From the dimensions of Gullstrand's schematic eye, the entrance pupil is approximately 0.5mm closer to us and about 14% larger than the real pupil (Figure 1). Because the entrance pupil is conjugate to the real pupil, light rays directed toward the entrance pupil will be refracted by the cornea and will pass through the actual pupil.

Light rays from a point fixated by the patient fall upon the entire eye, but only that bundle of rays bounded by the entrance pupil will enter the eye. Consequently, the only portion of the cornea used to see the fixation point is the portion that overlies the entrance pupil and is centered on the line connecting the fixation point with the center of the entrance pupil. This line is called the "line of sight," corresponding in geometrical optics terms to the chief ray of the bundle of rays reaching the fovea. For best optical performance, therefore, it is the intersection of the line of sight with the cornea that marks the desired center for the optical zone of corneal surgical procedures.

Table 1
Diameter of Clear Optical Zone for
Glare-Free Distance Vision (mm)*

Visual Field Radius	Entrance Pupil Diameter (mm)					
(degrees)	**2.00**	**3.00**	**4.00**	**5.00**	**6.00**	**7.00**
0 (fixation point only)	2.00	3.00	4.00	5.00	6.00	7.00
5	2.52	3.50	4.48	5.45	6.41	7.37
15	3.53	4.46	5.38	6.28	7.17	8.04
30	5.04	5.86	6.66	7.43	8.18	8.91
45	6.62	7.29	7.93	8.55	9.14	9.71
60	8.36	8.83	9.27	9.70	10.12	10.51

If this optical zone is too small or is not centered properly, irregular astigmatism and glare can seriously interfere with visual function.

For a patient to have a zone of glare-free vision centered on the point of fixation, the optical zone of the cornea must be larger than the entrance pupil. The larger the optical zone, the larger the field of glare-free vision (Table 1). No matter how large the optical zone of the cornea, it must still be centered on the line of sight if the zone of glare-free vision is to be centered about the fixation point.

The natural pupil is optimally used for centering corneal surgical procedures, because medications used to dilate or constrict the pupil can sometimes shift its center.

If the geometric center is used, however, and the pupil is markedly eccentric, glare will result. If the glare is primarily in the peripheral visual field, it may be tolerable. Fortunately, most pupils are close enough to the geometric center of the cornea that centering the corneal surgical procedure on the line of sight causes no problem with wound healing.

An argument might be made that proper centering should take into account the Stiles-Crawford effect: because the photoreceptors are aimed toward the center of the normal pupil, light passing through the center of the pupil is more effective in stimulating the photoreceptors than light passing through the peripheral pupil. With eccentric pupils, Enoch and Laties' and Bonds and MacLeod have demonstrated that the photoreceptors actively orient themselves toward the center of the eccentric pupil. Therefore, the pupil remains the proper optical reference for centering corneal surgical procedures.

The Corneal Light Reflex

The corneal light reflex is often used for centering, but its actual location is not widely understood. Many surgeons believe it is on the cornea, in the anterior chamber, or in the plane of the entrance pupil. Based on calculations from Gullstrand's schematic eye, it is actually about 0.85 mm posterior to the plane of the entrance pupil.

The location of the corneal light reflex, however, is not constant.

Table 2
Centering Error With Osher's Centering Device (mm)*

Working Distance (mm)	Angle Lambda (λ)			
	3 Degrees	4 Degrees	5 Degrees	6 Degrees
150	0.237	0.316	0.395	0.475
175	0.238	0.318	0.398	0.478
200	0.240	0.320	0.401	0.481

* Calculated for customary working distances of the operating microscope and for various normal values of the angle lambda.

Table 3
Worse-Case Centering Error With the Zeiss
or Weck Fixation Device (mm)*

Working Distance (mm)	Angle Lambda (λ)			
	3 Degrees	4 Degrees	5 Degrees	6 Degrees
150	0.553	0.631	0.710	0.789
(-0.008)	(-0.001)	(-0.078)	(0.157)	
175	0.518	0.597	0.677	0.756
(-0.042)	(0.038)	(0.117)	(0.196)	
200	0.478	0.558	0.638	0.717
(0.001)	(0.080)	(0.160)	(0.240)	

* If the surgeon uses his right eye for sighting the patient's right eye, and his left eye only for sighting the patient's left eye, the centering error is much less, as given by the values in parentheses.

Table 4
Centering Error When Sighting Monocularly with
Thornton's Fixation Target

Working Distance (mm)	Centering Error (mm)
150	0.249
175	0.214
200	0.188

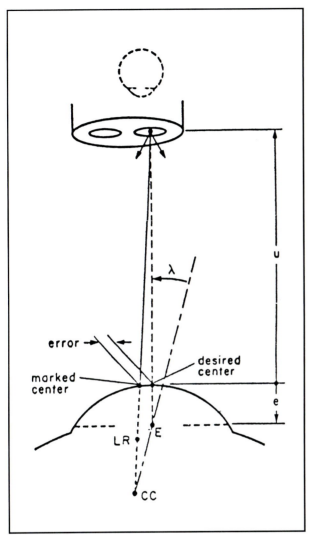

Figure 2. (Uozato and Guyton). Schematic illustration of the error in corneal centering produced by Osher's Optical Centering Device. The fixation light is centered in one viewing tube of the operating microscope. The other viewing tube is covered. If the center of the entrance pupil (E) were used for sighting, rather than the corneal light reflex (LR), the desired center would be localized.

Current Methods of Corneal Centering

Various methods have been described for centering corneal surgical procedures with operating microscope. Steinberg and Waring sight the corneal light reflex monocularly through one side of the microscope. The main illumination lamp of the microscope serves as the light source, which the patient is asked to fixate. Because the light source is not coaxial with the examiner's line of sight, the intersection of the visual axis with the cornea is estimated and marked as being displaced a designated amount from the apparent position of the corneal light reflex. Using this method, error can result from the patient's not fixing the center of the light source, from the offset estimation required of the surgeon, and from the use of the corneal light reflex in the first place.

Several arrangements have been described to decrease the potential error from

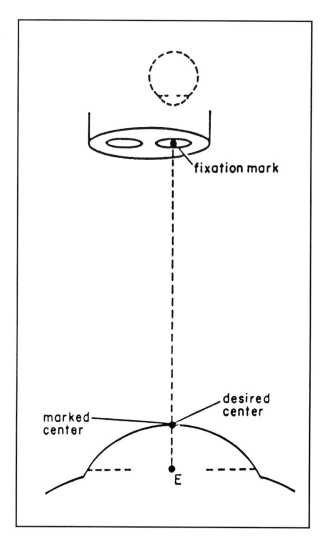

Figure 3. (Uozato and Guyton). Optimal corneal centering. The patient sights a fixation mark placed in the center of one of the viewing tubes of the microscope, and the surgeon views monocularly through that tube and marks the patient's cornea in line with the center of the entrance pupil.

such non-coaxial sighting by the examiner. Osher's Optical Centering Device (JEDMED Instrument Co.) covers over the main illumination system but channels some of the light to emerge from a sport in the exact center of one of the viewing tubes of the microscope. The patient fixates the spot of light, the examiner views monocularly through the viewing tube, and the visual axis is marked as coinciding with the apparent position of the corneal light reflex. A second arrangement has recently been added to the Weck operating microscope (Weck Surgical Systems) and as an attachment to the Zeiss microscope (Carl Zeiss, Inc.). A fixation light is added to the microscope exactly between the two viewing tubes. The patient fixates the light, and the examiner sights the corneal light reflex of the fixation light binocularly, marking its apparent position as the visual axis. A third arrangement, described by Thornton, uses a nonluminous fixation target mounted exactly between the two viewing tubes of the microscope. The patient fixates the target, and the examiner sights binocularly to mark the center of the pupil.

Binocular sighting—Centering methods using binocular sighting have been based on the assumption that binocular sighting is valid. Experiments showed that approximately one sixth of the surgeons sighted monocularly, approximately one half binocularly, and the remaining one third somewhere in between.

Only half of the surgeons who sighted monocularly were aware that they customarily did so. Monocular sighting leads to centering errors in those techniques that rely on binocular sighting. By looking first with one eye and then with the other, most monocular sighters could learn to balance the position of corneal line of sight.

Techniques for Optimal Corneal Centering

Thornton's fixation target—With Thornton's fixation target, a centering error arises only when the surgeon does not sight binocularly. The fixation target is placed midway between the two viewing tubes, coaxial with neither (Figure 2). In the case of monocular sighting, the error can be derived (Table 4). The error is approximately 0.2 mm in all cases, assuming the viewing tubes are 25 mm between centers.

While centering errors of 0.2 mm are not significant clinically, errors of 0.5 to 0.8 mm can be, especially with scarfree optical zones of only 2.5 to 3.0 mm in diameter.

Weck and Zeiss fixation lights—With either the Weck or the Zeiss fixation light, the surgeon sights the corneal light reflex of the fixation light (Figure 3). Centering error results not only from the angle lambda in sighting the corneal light reflex, but also if the surgeon sights monocularly, for the fixation light is not coaxial with either viewing tube (Table 3).

The corneal light reflex should not be used, however, because of error arising from the angle lambda. The center of the patient's entrance pupil is the proper sighting point, not the corneal light reflex.

The operating microscope can be used without Osher's device if a fixation spot is placed in the exact center of one of the viewing tubes of the microscope (Figure 4). A 1- or 2-mm mark will not interfere significantly with the optics. The surgeon should sight monocularly through the tube with the fixation spot and mark the cornea at the center of the patient's entrance pupil.

Optimal corneal centering requires the patient to have a natural pupil and to fixate on a light or target that is coaxial with the examiner's sighting eye.

References

1. Walsh PM, and Guyton DL: Comparison of two methods of marking the visual axis on the cornea during radial keratotomy. *Am J Ophthalmol* 1984, 97:660.

2. Bennett AG, and Francis JL: The eye as an optical system. In Davson, H. (ed.): *The Eye*. New York Academic Press, 1962, 4: 101.

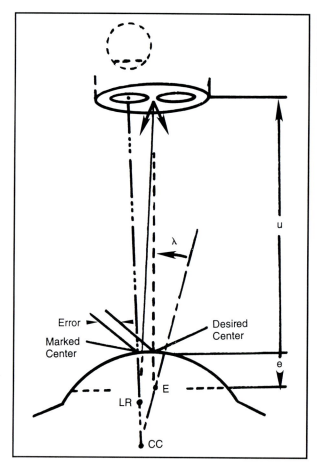

Figure 4. (Uozato and Guyton). Schematic illustration of the maximum error in corneal centering caused by monocular sighting of the corneal light reflex as the patient fixates the Zeiss or Weck fixation device.

3. Fry GA: *Geometrical Optics*. Philadelphia, Chilton, 1969, 110.

4. Enoch JM, and Laties AM: An analysis of retinal receptor orientation. II. Prediction for psychophysical tests. *Invest. Ophthalmol* 1971, 10:959.

5. Bonds AB, and MacLeod DIA: A displaced Stiles-Crawford effect associated with an eccentric pupil. *Invest. Ophthalmol. Vis. Sci.* 1978, 17:754.

6. Lancaster WB: Terminology in ocular motility and allied subjects. *Am J Ophthalmol* 1943, 26:122.

7. Uozato H, Makino H, Saishin M, and Nakao S: Measurement of visual axis using a laser beam. In Breinin GM, and Siegel IM (eds): Advances in Diagnostic Visual Optics. Berlin, Springer-Verlag, 1983, 22.

8. Steinberg EB, and Waring GO III: Comparison of two methods of marking the visual axis on the cornea during radial keratotomy. Am J Ophthalmol. 1983, 96:605.

9. Thornton SP: Surgical armamentarium. In Sanders DR, Hofmann RF, and Salz JJ (eds): *Refractive Corneal Surgery*. Thorofare, New Jersey, SLACK Inc., 1986, 134.

Appendix C

Sample Forms and Letters

The sample letters and forms in the following pages have been developed to provide information for patients, families, and other concerned individuals and agencies. They can be adapted to any type of practice and any type of surgery.

We have found it helpful to have some letters to patients and insurance companies sent out under the signature of the nurse assistant or secretary in order to allow the physician to be shielded from unnecessary phone calls and correspondence which can easily be handled by staff.

Here are some sample patient information letters, letters to insurance companies, evaluation forms, consent forms, and pre-operative and intra-operative forms. Feel free to modify them for your own office.

Dear Patient:

Please forgive me for sending a form letter in answer to your request, but the number of inquiries we receive makes it difficult to answer each one personally. I assure you that Dr. Thornton is personally interested in you, and if at all possible, he will try to help you. The enclosed forms should be filled out and returned to us at the above address. They will provide us with the information to enable us to evaluate your condition.

The surgery to correct nearsightedness and some types of astigmatism was developed in the 1970s by a Russian ophthalmologist, Dr. S.N. Fyodorov, at the Moscow Institute of Clinical Eye Surgery. After performing this operation for a number of years and helping thousands of patients, Dr. Fyodorov reported a success rate of over 85%. Currently about 75,000 operations are performed each year in the United States by American ophthalmologists with a success rate of over 95%. Dr. Thornton was one of the first ophthalmologists in America to perform this surgery and is internationally recognized for his expertise and experience with this operation. Since this is still a relatively new concept in surgery, it is being conducted under what is known as a clinical investigation plan. With any new surgery, we feel that patients should be followed from time to time either in our office, or the office of the patient's own eye doctor if they live a distance away. If needed, we will assist the patient in locating a qualified eye doctor to continue postoperative care in their own area.

The preoperative evaluation of the patient is important not only to insure proper preparation for the operation, but also to enable the doctor to decide if a person's eye is suitable for the operation. Preoperatively, in addition to a thorough external and internal eye examination, special tests are done, such as: keratotomy (measuring the curvature of the front of the cornea of the eye), pachymetry (measuring the thickness of the different parts of the cornea where incisions will be made), corneal size measurements, evaluation of the corneal endothelium, ultrasound measurements of the length and size of the eye, etc.

Let me describe various aspects of the operation. The cornea is the clear cover of the eye which is in front of the iris (colored part of the eye). Based on calculations from the preoperative tests and measurements, special incisions are made into, not through the cornea. This is performed under the operating microscope and is called microsurgery. These incisions change the shape of the cornea and thus eliminate or reduce the nearsightedness. The inside of the eye is not usually entered by this operation on the cornea.

One eye is done at a time and only local anesthesia is used. Patients who are extremely anxious or nervous can be given a short-acting medication. The operation takes only about twenty minutes after which a patch is put over the eye. The operation is done on an outpatient basis and the patient may leave shortly thereafter.

The improvement in vision usually begins a short time after removal of the eye patch and continues for the next several weeks. There will be variation of vision during the first several months of healing. This usually moderates between four to six weeks, but may persist for several months. Also, postoperatively some patients report glare, especially at night. This usually diminishes after four to six weeks.

It is important to know that this revolutionary operation is for correction of nearsightedness and astigmatism. It does not treat glaucoma or cataracts, or other illnesses which affect and damage vision. It cannot make a blind eye see. If an eye can see with glasses or contact lenses, the operation can help that eye to see better without the glasses or contact lenses. If a person is happy with this present method of correction (glasses or contact lenses), he or she should by all means continue with it.

This operation is an alternative for those who wish to dispense with their glasses or contact lenses, and for those who cannot pursue certain careers and professions because they are not permitted to wear glasses or contact lenses.

As with any new procedure in medicine, there will be a certain amount of positive and negative criticism from within the medical profession. You, the patient, must evaluate the validity of these comments. I have studied and assisted Dr. Thornton in performing the operation many times and we have taught many eye surgeons how to perform it. If you feel it is necessary, you can certainly consult other ophthalmologists for their opinions.

Reputable ophthalmologists may disagree concerning the safety and efficacy of radial keratotomy for nearsightedness. Skepticism in the profession of medicine in the evaluation of new techniques is healthy. However, I might mention that years ago doctors were critical of those who performed intraocular lens implantation for patients with cataracts. As the critics saw the results and learned to perform the operation themselves, many of them joined the ranks of the "do-ers." Today, intraocular lens implantation is recognized by most as the best way to help the cataract patient. We feel essentially the same will happen as more doctors learn and perform this new procedure to correct nearsightedness.

It is my understanding that medical expenses, including travel expenses in relation to medical care, are tax deductible. For patients who wish to come to Nashville from other cities, we can recommend local accommodations.

As I previously mentioned, if you are interested in the operation, please complete the enclosed forms and return them to our office where we will make a preliminary evaluation as to the possibility of you being a candidate for the surgery.

I hope this letter has answered most of your questions. If there are any further questions, please feel free to call or write our office.

Sincerely yours,

Jean S. Robertson, RN, COT
Assistant to Dr. Thornton

Preliminary Evaluation Form for Refractive Surgery

Name _____ Age glasses first worn _____

Date glasses last changed _____ Eye Doctor _____

Occupation _____

The following information will help us make a preliminary determination of your eligibility for surgery. Please obtain this information from your eye doctor or optician.

Prescription of glasses: Right _____ Left _____

Keratometry Readings: Right _____ Left _____

Ever worn contact lenses? No Yes What type? Hard Soft

What problems have you had with contacts?

Discomfort _____ Vision not as good at night _____

Glare _____ Frequent irritation _____

Intolerance to lenses _____ Eyes dry or burn _____

Recurrent abrasions of cornea _____

Note: Hard contact lenses must not be worn for three weeks prior to your office evaluation.
   Soft contact lenses must not be worn for one week prior to your office evaluation.

What problems have you had with glasses?

Side vision blocked _____ Uncomfortable _____

Hard to adjust _____ Other _____

Hard to keep clean _____ _____

Any allergies? No Yes To What? _____

On birth control pills or any medications? No Yes

For what conditions? _____

Any history of eye injury? No Yes Any infections? No Yes

Why are you interested in refractive surgery (surgical reduction of myopia/astigmatism)?

_____

_____

_____

Since the long-term risks and benefits of Radial/Astigmatic Keratotomy have not been conclusively determined, do you wish to participate in what may be considered non-standard treatment for myopia and astigmatism? Yes No

Signed _____ Date _____

Please return the Patient Registration Form along with this Preliminary Evaluation Form to Dr. Thornton at 2010 Church Street, #307 Nashville TN 37203. The secretary will call or write to set up an appointment for your initial examination if we feel you are a candidate for the surgery.

Questions on Radial Keratotomy Preparing for Surgery Video

(1993, Patient Education Concepts, Houston, Texas)

Print your name: ————————————————   Date: ————————————————

The following questions cover important information contained in the video presentation. Please mark the correct answer. If you need more time to answer a question than the video presentation allows, skip that question and return to it when the program is over.

1. TRUE OR FALSE: RK surgery will permanently change the shape of my cornea.

2. TRUE OR FALSE: Modern equipment and surgical techniques have greatly improved your doctor's ability to perform RK, but there are no guarantees as to exactly how well you will see after the procedure.

3. TRUE OR FALSE: RK is not the only way to correct your nearsightedness. You can still wear corrective lenses as an alternative to RK surgery.

4. TRUE OR FALSE: You may experience vision irregularities such as halos or starbursts around lights after your surgery, and in rare cases they may be permanent.

5. TRUE OR FALSE: After the surgery, the eye can be more easily damaged by direct blow.

6. TRUE OR FALSE: RK carries certain risks including infection and loss of vision.

7. TRUE OR FALSE: RK is considered to be cosmetic surgery.

8. TRUE OR FALSE: RK will eliminate your need to wear reading glasses when you are over 40 years of age.

9. TRUE OR FALSE: It may be necessary to "enhance" or "fine tune" my surgery with additional procedures.

10. TRUE OR FALSE: This video program covered all risks, side-effects and complications that could possibly occur with RK surgery.

Please check your answers with the correct answers below. Mark any that you missed. If you are still unsure as to why you missed any of these questions, take the form to the doctor or staff member for an explanation.

ANSWERS:
1. *True.* The purpose of RK is to permanently change the shape of the cornea.
2. *True.* There are no guarantees as to how well you will see after RK.
3. *True.* RK surgery is an alternative to either glasses or contacts which can, in most cases, provide you with useful vision.
4. *True.* These side-effects have been reported and occasionally can be permanent.
5. *True.* Some studies show that direct blows to RK eyes can cause more damage than the same blow to an unoperated eye.
6. *True.* Although extremely remote, infection and vision loss are potential risks of RK surgery.
7. *False.* RK is not cosmetic surgery. Because its aim is to provide better visual function, it is considered functional surgery.
8. *False.* RK does not correct the condition known as presbyopia which occurs to most people above age 40 and requires them to wear reading glasses for close work.
9. *True.* It may be possible or necessary to have additional surgery to "enhance" or "fine tune" the initial result.
10. *False.* The video did not cover all possible risks, side-effects and complications.

Use this space to write any questions or concerns you still wish to ask the doctor or a staff member and be sure they are answered to your satisfaction.

——

——

——

——

Consent to Have RK Surgery

This information is to help you make an informed decision about having Radial Keratotomy surgery to correct your nearsightedness and/or astigmatism. Take as much time as you wish to make a decision about signing this form. You are encouraged to ask any questions and have them answered to your satisfaction before you give your permission for surgery. Every surgery has risks as well as benefits and each person must evaluate this risk/benefit ratio for him/herself in light of the information presented in the video and the information which follows.

1) RK permanently changes the shape of the cornea as a result of making a number of incisions around the center of the eye. This causes the center of the cornea to flatten, which changes the focusing power of the cornea. Although the goal of RK is to improve vision to the point of not wearing glasses, or to the point of wearing thinner (or weaker) glasses, this result is not guaranteed. Incisions in any surgery cause scarring, and RK is no exception. These scars are not usually visible to the naked eye but are permanent and visible with magnification.

2) RK surgery to correct nearsightedness and astigmatism can possibly cause loss of vision or loss of best corrected vision. This can be due to infection or irregular scaring or other causes, and unless successfully controlled by antibiotics or other necessary treatment, could even cause loss of the infected eye. Vision loss can be due to the cornea healing irregularly which could add astigmatism and make wearing glasses or contact lenses necessary and useful vision could also be lost.

3) It may be that RK surgery will not give you the result you desired. Many procedures result in the eye being undercorrected in which case, it may be possible or necessary to have additional surgery to "fine tune" or "enhance" the initial result. These results cannot be guaranteed. It is also possible that your eye may be overcorrected to the point of remaining farsighted.

4) RK does not correct the condition known as presbyopia (or aging of the eye) which occurs in most people around age forty and requires them to wear reading glasses for close-up work. People over 40 that have their nearsightedness corrected may have presbyopia induced by the procedure which would necessitate the use of reading glasses.

5) Other complications and conditions that can occur with RK surgery include: anisometropia (difference in power between the two eyes); aniseikonia (difference in image size between the two eyes); double vision; corneal perforation which could possibly require sutures; incisional inclusions; corneal vascularization; corneal ulcer formation; endothelial cell loss, epithelial healing defects; cataract formation; fluctuating vision during the day and from day to day; increased sensitivity to light which may be incapacitating for some time and may not completely go away, and glare and halos around lights which may not completely go away. Some of these conditions may affect your ability to drive and judge distances and driving should only be done when you are certain your vision is adequate.

6) You should understand that RK surgery will not prevent you from developing naturally occurring eye problems such as glaucoma, cataracts, retinal degeneration or detachment. You should also be aware that your eye will be more susceptible to traumatic blow to the globe during the healing phase, and possibly somewhat after healing as the microscopic scar tissue may not be as strong as normal tissue. It is also possible that your cornea could continue to flatten over a period of years to the point that you would become farsighted.

7) You should also be aware that there are other complications that could occur that were not reported prior to the creation of this consent form, as RK surgery has been performed in the United States only since 1979 and longer term results may reveal additional risks and complications. There are also potential complications due to anesthesia and medications which may involve other parts of your body. Since it is impossible to state all potential risks of any surgery, this form is incomplete.

8) In signing this form, you are stating that you have read this consent form and although it contains medical terms which you may not completely understand, you have had the opportunity to ask questions and had them answered to your satisfaction. You have also viewed the video and understand the questions presented on the other side of this form.

9) You also give your permission for medical data concerning your operation and related treatment and any video recordings of your surgery to be released to physicians and others demonstrating a "need to know" for clinical study.

I am making an informed decision in giving my permission to have Radial Keratotomy and/or Astigmatic Keratotomy surgery performed on my eye(s) to correct my nearsightedness and/or astigmatism.

Signature of Patient: _____   Date: _____

Signature of Witness: _____   Date: _____

Signature of Surgeon: _____   Date: _____

ATTN: Benefits Determination

RE:

Your above named insured has asked us to write to you regarding radial and/or astigmatic keratotomy, a form of refractive surgery, which he/she wishes to have performed on his/her eyes. Recent reports indicate that an estimated 150,000 cases per year are done around the world, about 75,000 in the U.S. by American doctors.

The surgery involves making specially-designed incisions into the peripheral cornea in order to change the shape of the cornea and thus eliminate or reduce the nearsightedness and/or astigmatism. This is performed under a high power operating microscope.

One eye is done at a time. In most cases, only local anesthesia is used. The operation is done in the out-patient surgery center operating room and takes approximately twenty minutes, after which a bandage is placed over the eye. The patient can go home immediately after surgery and the bandage is removed the next day.

This operation requires extensive and sophisticated evaluation of the corneas. It requires special preoperative tests such as keratometry (measuring the curvature of the front of the eye), pachymetry (measuring the thickness of the different parts of the cornea where the incisions will be made), corneal size measurements, length of the eye, and computer analysis.

This operation is designed to help individuals who have difficulty wearing glasses or contact lenses and is an alternative method of treatment for myopia and astigmatism. The current surgical fee for this procedure is _____ per eye; preoperative evaluation is _____; and the approximate surgery center charges would be around _____ per eye. If you have any further questions about this surgery please do not hesitate to call.

Sincerely yours,

Jean S. Robertson, RN, COT
Assistant to Spencer P. Thornton, MD

Insurance Co.
Chicago, IL

ATTN: Benefits Determination Dept.

RE: John Joseph Smith 8721369241

Dear Sir or Madam,

John Joseph Smith was examined in my office today because of visual difficulties he has experienced since age seven. His uncorrected visual acuity of finger counting in both eyes makes him totally dependent on corrective lenses. His experience with contact lenses and glasses, however, has been unsatisfactory. Contact lenses have caused frequent irritation, dryness and burning. Glasses do not provide adequate peripheral vision. These difficulties are complicated by the progressive nature of his myopia and astigmatism. His refractive error upon examination today was OD -6.75 -0.50 x 115 and OS -6.25 -0.75 x 165 compared to -6.00 sphere OU just one year ago.

Because of his visual difficulties Mr. Smith would like to have radial keratotomy eye surgery for correction of his myopia and astigmatism. He has tried contact lenses and glasses and these alternatives have not been satisfactory. Therefore, he has requested corrective eye surgery. Also, Mr. Smith's desired occupation in law enforcement will be unattainable without better visual acuity.

As a surgeon specializing in refractive surgery, I am very selective in choosing patients for radial keratotomy eye surgery. In Mr. Smith's case, I believe he would be a suitable candidate for this procedure. Also, because of his visual history and his planned occupation, I recommend radial keratotomy as a medical and an occupational necessity in his case.

Please let us know what benefits are available.

Sincerely,

Spencer P. Thornton, MD, FACS

Preparing for Astigmatic and/or Radial Keratotomy

Jean S. Robertson, RN, COT
Assistant to Dr. Thornton

Now that you are planning to have astigmatic or radial keratotomy surgery there are some more instructions we need to give you. These will help you to prepare for your surgery as well as care for yourself after your surgery.

If you wear hard contact lenses, leave the contacts out of the eye for three weeks prior to your surgery; for soft contact lenses, leave them out for one week. We want your eye to be free from any irritation and induced changes from the contacts. If you wear glasses, you might want to check with your optical shop preoperatively to make arrangements for a lens without power to be put in your glasses after surgery.

Three days prior to surgery, women need to take special care to remove all eye make-up from the eye you are preparing for surgery. Even when you are very careful in removing eye make-up, fine particles are usually left and can be seen under magnification. This is why we ask you to avoid eye make-up for this period prior to surgery.

To help prepare your eye for surgery, you will need to use some antibiotic eyedrops. Put one drop in your operative eye four times on the day before surgery. Then, the morning of surgery, put one drop in when you first get up and repeat before coming to the office. Please remember to wash your hands each time before using the drops and always shake the bottle. Please bring these drops with you when you return to the office the day after surgery so that we can put them in after removing your bandage.

You will need to make arrangements to get to the office by the time we have indicated. Also, make arrangements for someone to drive you home after surgery. Something else you might want to do before surgery is get an ice pack or some zip lock bags to use as a cold pack after surgery.

On the day of your surgery, do not eat your usual breakfast. You may have only orange juice and a piece of toast unless we tell you otherwise. Do not drink any coffee, tea, colas, or anything else after your juice and toast. Don't drink anything with caffeine for 24 hours prior to your surgery.

Please wear a short-sleeved garment to the office the day of surgery, preferably something that buttons up the front.

When you get to the office, you will be checked in and taken to a preparation area. Here you will be asked to put on a hospital gown and shoe covers over your clothes and shoes and remove all jewelry except your wedding band (if you wish to leave it on). You may wish to leave your jewelry at home.

Next, medications will be given to prepare you for surgery. You will be given a pill to help you relax. You may feel sleepy from this medication and this is fine, just relax.

When you are taken to the operating area, we will put several drops in your eye and Dr. Thornton will examine your cornea under the microscope and mark the exact center of the pupil. You will not feel any pain or discomfort from your surgery, although you may be aware that we are moving or touching your eye. The surgery itself will not last long (usually only 15 or 20 minutes). When finished, we will put a pressure bandage on your eye and take you back to the preparation area. Here you can relax and you will be given a prescription for pain medication to have filled on the way home.

When you go home, you will do better if you keep both eyes closed as much as possible, because even with a bandage on your eye you will have movement under the lid if you move the unbandaged eye. Also, place the ice pack or ice filled baggie over the bandage. This will aid in your comfort. Take your pain medication as directed if needed.

During this time you may notice that your eye feels like it is tearing under your bandage. This is normal, but do not loosen your bandage unless instructed to do so by Dr. Thornton. We will remove the bandage in the office the next day.

The day following surgery, you will return to the office to have your eye examined under the microscope. You will need to bring your eyedrops with you at this time. We will start the drops after examining your eye and you will continue these drops four times a day until they are used up unless instructed otherwise.

You might want to bring sunglasses with you. We can give you a pair of sunglasses in the office if you need some the day following surgery. As pointed out in the videotape, you might be sensitive to sunlight immediately after surgery. Glare, either at night or in the sunlight, might be noticed postoperatively. As your eye heals, this should gradually disappear.

Another thing you should expect is fluctuation of vision. This means that you may see great one day and poorly the next, or good in the morning and poorly in the evening. Do not be alarmed by this when it occurs, and it probably will, even if it is not evident immediately after surgery. Sometimes this may be noticed several months after surgery.

You should expect to have some swelling (puffiness) of your eyelids when the bandage is removed. Some bruising occurs in a small number of patients. Also, you eye will probably be somewhat red. Do not let any of this worry you. All of this begins to subside soon. However, do not try to cover this up with eye make-up.

During the time immediately postoperatively, you can do just about anything you want with a few restrictions. Most important: DO NOT RUB YOUR EYE. You may use your eye as much as you want, even though it may feel like it gets tired or your eyes are competing. It will not harm your eyes but this may require some patience on your part. As far as physical activity, you are not restricted; however, do be careful the first week after surgery. Be careful when washing your face or hair not to get soap or shampoo in your eyes. Likewise, it is better to avoid swimming for a week after surgery. If you play any contact sports, wear some sort of protective glasses for a few weeks after surgery.

If you have any questions about any of this material or anything not covered here please let us know. Also, after your surgery, let us know if you have any problems. We don't mind you calling us at any time.

Pre-Operative Instructions for Outpatient Surgery Patients

We have scheduled your surgery for _____ at our surgery facility. You will need to report to the office by _____ on this day.

1. Follow the preoperative instruction booklet given to you to prepare for surgery. Please remember to use your eyedrops in your_____ eye the day before surgery and the morning of your surgery.

2. On the morning of surgery you may have orange juice and toast. No coffee or caffeine products 24 hours prior to surgery.

Please tell your family that Dr. Thornton would like to talk with them after your surgery. He will give them instructions about postoperative activities and precautions.

After your surgery you will be taken back to the preparation area where you may begin to be up and around. You may feel the effects of sedation so you may need help in preparing to go home but you are not limited to bed rest. You will be able to leave shortly after surgery.

You will return to the office the day after your surgery. Dr. Thornton will tell you what time to come. You will need to have someone drive you to and from the office.

We hope this helps you understand more about what to expect. There is always some anxiety in preparing for surgery and sometimes there are questions that you forget or are hesitant to ask. Please know that Dr. Thornton and his staff are concerned in every way for your well-being and do not mind you asking about anything that worries you. We want you to have the best care, and if there is any way that we can make you more comfortable, please let us know.

Radial/Astigmatic Keratotomy

Name _____ Date _____ Patient # _____

Pre-Op Orders

1. For RK/AK
2. Valium 10 mg PO 30 min. prior to SG

Post-Op Orders

1. Valium 5 mg po q 6 h #16 (Rx given)
2. Vistaril 50 mg po q 4 h PRN #20 (Rx given)
3. Usual Diet
4. Discharge when stable

History

This patient is admitted for surgical correction of myopia/astigmatism_____.
This patient desires surgical correction due to general incumbrances of wearing a significant spectacle correction. Contact lenses have/have not been worn in the past successfully/unsuccessfully (failure due to poor comfort/poor vision).

On examination, the patient was found to have uncorrected VA of _____ and best corrected acuity of _____ with a correction of _____ . External examination, pupil, motility, confrontation fields, slit lamp examinations and funcoscopic examination by indirect ophthalmoscopy were normal with the following exceptions.

_____

Impression:_____ Myopia _____Astigmatism _____

Allergies: _____

Current Medications: _____

Plan: _____

_____

Date _____

Operative Procedure

Name _____   Date _____

Patient # _____

Pre-Op Diagnosis: _____ myopia   _____ astigmatism

Operative Procedure: _____ Radial _____ Astigmatic Keratotomy

Surgeon: Spencer P. Thornton, MD   Assistant: Jean S. Robertson, RN, COT

Anesthesia: Topical   Anesthetic: 2% Xylocaine

Procedure: The patient was prepped and draped for sterile field, exposing the
_____ eye, and the optical center carefully marked under the microscope. A lid
speculum was introduced. The _____ mm optical zone marker was used to
mark the central optical zone centered on the visual axis mark. _____ radial
incisions were carried from the optical zone to the limbus and carried to the depth
of _____ microns. T incisions were made as follows: _____
_____

The incisions were carefully irrigated, inspected and found to be in good
condition. A sterile compress dressing was applied and the patient was taken from
the operating room in good condition.

_____

Spencer P. Thornton, MD

Name _____

Date _____

Blade Depth	Position	Blade Type	OZ	Perforation Location	Unusual Conditions

Eye _____

Note: Standard position numbering used: based on 16 radials, no. 16 = 12 o'clock, numbered clockwise.

Radial Keratotomy Evaluation Form

Name _____ DOB _____ Date _____

VA s Rx: OD 20/ OS 20/   VA c Rx: OD 20/ OS 20/   Dominant Eye _____

Last Rx: Date _____   OD ___−___ × ___   OS ___−___ × ___

Current Refraction in − Cyl form   OD ___−___ × ___   OS ___−___ × ___

Spherical Equivalent   OD _____   OS _____

Keratometry (Automatic)   OD ___×___ / ___×___   OS ___×___ / ___×___

Keratometry (Manual)   OD ___×___ / ___×___   OS ___×___ / ___×___

IOP: OD ___ OS ___   Diameter: OD ___ OS ___   Axial Length: OD___ OS___

OD   PACHYMETRY   OS

3mm Avg _____   3mm Avg _____

5mm Avg _____   5mm Avg _____

7mm Avg _____   7mm Avg _____

Age ___ Sex ___ = ± % _____   OD Working Sphere _____ OS Working Sphere _____

IOP, Pach, Diam, AvgK = ± % _____   OD Working Cylinder _____ OS Working Cylinder _____

Total Sph Modifier % = ± % _____

Cyl Modifier % (1/4 Sph) = ± % _____

OD: OZ _____ mm No._____   OS: OZ _____ mm No._____

Blade setting _____ μ   Blade setting _____ μ

Redeepen @ 5 to _____ μ @ 7 to_____ μ   Redeepen @ 5 to _____ μ @ 7 to_____ μ

___ "T" Incisions_____ °Axis _____ °Depth _____ μ   ___ "T" Incisions_____ °Axis _____ °Depth _____ μ

Appendix D

Trouble-Shooters Guide

I Didn't Get The Result I Wanted. Why?

Look for equipment errors, measurement errors, calculation errors, technique errors, and unforeseen biological errors.

1. Equipment errors

   a. Micrometer knife handles may give incorrect readings (check with microscope).

   b. Pachymeter may give incorrect readings (use test block periodically).

   c. Keratometer may give improper or incorrect readings (compare with topography).

   d. Eye not firm enough and incisions shallow (use Thornton Fixation Ring).

2. Measurement errors

   a. Non-cycloplegic refraction.

   b. Pachymetry done at wrong places or improperly done.

   c. Keratometry not confirmed with topography.

3. Calculation errors

   Any "simplified" method which ignores modifiers and employs "short-cuts" which eliminate necessary steps in calculation may result in errors. It is imperative to calculate the errors in plus cylinder *and* minus cylinder form as well as the spherical equivalent in *all cases* (for practice even if not needed in any one particular case).

As a safeguard, have a trusted assistant work out the formulas separately, then compare.

If the determination of optical zone sizes by calculating the effect of modifiers does not appeal to you because of its complexity, you can rely on available computer programs which contain the nomograms for correction of myopia and astigmatism.

4. Technical errors
   Too much pressure, too little pressure, improper fixation.

5. Unforseen biological errors
   Under and over-responses related to unforseeable biological variables. These variables must be considered in planning subsequent procedures.

Appendix E

Recommended Reading

For the serious student of refractive surgery I recommend the following books and journal articles for a deeper understanding of the field.

Refractive Corneal Surgery, edited by Donald R. Sanders, Robert F. Hofmann and James J. Salz, Thorofare, NJ, SLACK Incorporated, 1986. With twenty-seven authors contributing in their areas of expertise, this book is a classic. Beginning with a look at the development of radial keratotomy, sections on patient selection, preoperative evaluation and surgical planning are followed by practical sections on predictability, surgical instrumentation and surgical technique. Postoperative management and complications are then covered with an authority that speaks from experience. The authors, experts all, do an excellent job of making this book both practical and authoritative.

Refractive Keratotomy for Myopia and Astigmatism, edited by George O. Waring III, St. Louis, MO, Mosby Year Book, 1992. This is a beautifully detailed book covering the entire field of incisional refractive surgery with extensive coverage of the history and development of refractive keratotomy from the nineteenth century to the present time. Waring draws from thirty-two experts to produce a book remarkable for its comprehensiveness and authority. The key sections authored by the experts are well illustrated and thoroughly documented. In my opinion, this is the definitive book in the field of refractive keratotomy.

Refractive Eye Surgery, by Leo D. Bores, Boston, Blackwell Scientific Publishers, 1993. This book was authored by the American who introduced radial keratotomy to the United States in 1978. Bores is uniquely qualified to present the background and theory of modern refractive surgery, and he does it with a keen sense of humor as well as a perceptive insight into the theory and clinical practice of modern incisional surgery. He covers the practical as well as the theoretical with the practicing surgeon in mind. The book is well illustrated and comprehensive. It is must reading for the well prepared refractive surgeon.

An Atlas of Corneal Topography, edited by Donald R. Sanders and Douglas D. Koch, Thorofare, NJ, SLACK Incorporated, 1993. Contributions from a number of highly recognized experts make this the most comprehensive publication on the subject. This excellently illustrated text documents and explains the breakthroughs in diagnosing and evaluating pathological conditions, and illustrates ways of planning and following surgical and laser procedures. The significance of corneal topography in detecting and managing postoperative complications is highlighted.

Journal of Cataract and Refractive Surgery: This is the official journal of the American Society of Cataract and Refractive Surgery. It carries articles of interest both to cataract and refractive surgeons and presents the best of the papers presented in ASCRS symposia in addition to current papers on state-of-the-art anterior segment surgery.

Journal of Refractive and Corneal Surgery: This is the official journal of the International Society of Refractive Keratoplasty, carrying articles of primary interest to the refractive surgeon. This journal is exclusively devoted to corneal surgery and deals with subjects of interest to the clinical refractive surgeon including new and experimental approaches to refractive surgery.

Chapter 2: Theory of Corneal Relaxing Incisions

Schachar RA, Black TD: *A Physicist's View of Radial Keratotomy: Keratorefraction*, 1980, Denison, TX, LAL Publishing, 195-220.

Fyodorov, SN, Agranovsky, AA: Long term results of anterior radial keratotomy, *J Ocul Ther Surg.* 217-223, July-Aug, 1982.

Thornton SP: Theory behind corneal relaxing incisions/Thornton Nomogram. In Gills JP, Martin RG, Sanders DR (eds): *Sutureless Cataract Surgery*. Thorofare, NJ, SLACK, 1992, 123-144.

Chapter 3: Patient Selection, Work-up and Informed Consent

Schachar RA, Black TD, Huang T: *Understanding Radial Keratotomy*. Denison, TX, LAL Publishing, 1981, 201-225.

Bores LD: Radial keratotomy: a progress report of the American experience. *Ophthalmic Forum.* 1:24-27, 1982.

Deitz MR: Patient Selection and Counseling. In Sanders DR, Hofmann RF, Salz JJ (eds): *Refractive Corneal Surgery*. Thorofare, NJ, SLACK, 1985, 35-48.

Hofmann RF: Preoperative Evaluation. In Sanders DR, Hofmann RF, Salz JJ (eds): *Refractive Corneal Surgery*. Thorofare, NJ, SLACK, 1985, 51-77.

Chapter 4: The Radial Keratotomy Nomogram

Thornton SP: Thornton guide for radial keratotomy incisions and optical zone size. *J Refract Surg*. 1985, 1:29-33.

Sanders DR, Deitz MR: Factors Affecting Predictability of Radial Keratotomy. In Sanders DR, Hofmann RF, Salz JJ (eds): *Refractive Corneal Surgery*, Thorofare, NJ, SLACK, 1985, 81-90.

Thornton SP: Radial keratotomy incisions and optical zone size. *J Greek IOI & Refract Surg Soc*. 1990, 3, 3, 57-63.

Sanders DR: Computerized Predictability Formulas for Refractive Keratotomy. In Waring GO (ed): *Refractive Keratotomy*, St. Louis, MO, Mosby Year Book, 1992, 381-401.

Chapter 5: Instruments for Refractive Surgery

Thornton SP: A new diamond blade configuration for transverse incisions. *Refract & Corneal Surg*. SLACK, Jan 1989, 5: 32.

Thornton SP: The double-V instrument block helps protect diamond blades. *Ocular Surg News*. SLACK, April 15, 1989, 32.

Thornton SP: Surgical maneuvers—a marker for length of relaxing incisions. *Ocular Surg News*. SLACK, April 1, 1989, 28.

Thornton SP: Report of the American Society of Cataract and Refractive Surgery International Committee on standards and quality control for ophthalmic instruments and devices. *J Cataract Refract Surg*. Baltimore, MD. Williams and Wilkins, 1993, 17, 359-365.

Thornton SP: Corneal press-on ruler for astigmatic keratotomy. *J Cataract Refract Surg*. Baltimore, MD. Williams and Wilkins, 5, Jan 1989, 96.

Allarakhia L, Thornton SP: Ophthalmic pre-inked marking pad. *J Cataract Refract Surg*. Baltimore, MD. Williams and Wilkins, 17, May 1991, 374.

Chapter 6: American vs. Russian Technique

Thornton SP: Cutting Instruments. In Sanders DR, Hofmann RF, Salz JJ (eds): *Refractive Corneal Surgery*, Thorofare, NJ, SLACK, 1985, 147-161.

Lewicky AO: Surgical Technique and Related Complications. In Sanders DR, Hofmann RF, Salz JJ (eds): *Refractive Corneal Surgery*, Thorofare, NJ, SLACK, 1985, 177-194.

Chapter 7: Blade Depth and Number of Incisions

Salz JJ: Pathophysiology of Radial and Astigmatic Keratotomy Incisions. In Sanders DR, Hofmann, RF, Salz JJ (eds), *Refractive Corneal Surgery*, Thorofare, NJ, SLACK, 1985, 111-127.

Sanders DR, (ed): *Radial Keratotomy—Surgical Techniques*, Thorofare, NJ, SLACK, 1986.

Chapter 8: Ocular Anesthesia

Thornton SP: Anesthesia for cataract surgery and its complications. *Current Opinion in Ophthal.* 1993, 4, 1:29-32.

Waring GO: Anesthetizing the Eye. In Waring, GO (ed) *Refractive Keratotomy*, St. Louis, MO, Mosby Year Book, 1992, 525-530.

Chapter 9: Determining the Visual Axis

Thornton SP: Binocular Method of Aligning and Marking the Visual Axis. Surgical Armamentarium. In Sanders DR, Hofmann RF, Salz JJ (eds): *Refractive Corneal Surgery*. Thorofare, NJ, SLACK, 1985, 134.

Uozato H, Guyton DL: Centering corneal surgical procedures. *Am J Ophthalmol.* Chicago, IL. Ophthalmic Publishing Co., 103:264-275, 1987.

Chapter 10: Astigmatic Keratotomy

Fenzl RE: Control of Astigmatism Using Corneal Incisions. In Sanders DR, Hofmann RF (eds): *Refractive Surgery: A Text of Radial Keratotomy*. Thorofare, NJ, SLACK, 1985, 151-166.

Thornton SP, Sanders DR: Graded nonintersecting transverse incisions for correction of idiopathic astigmatism. *J Cataract Refract Surg*. Jan 1987, 13:27-31.

Merlin U: Corneal keratotomy procedure for congenital astigmatism. *J Refract Surg*. 1987, 3:92-97.

Thornton SP: Current astigmatic keratotomy technique. *CLAO File*. Sept 1987, 2, 2:24.

Duffy RJ, Jain VN, Tchah, et al: Paired arcuate keratotomy: a surgical approach to mixed and myopic astigmatism. *Arch Ophthalmol*. Chicago, IL. American Medical Association, 1988, 106:1130-1135.

Thornton SP: Astigmatic keratotomy: a review of basic concepts with case reports. *J Cat Refract Surg*. Baltimore, MD. Williams and Wilkins, 1990, 16:430-435.

Thornton SP: Astigmatic keratotomy and the coupling phenomenon. *Ophthalmic Practice*. 1990, 8, 1:22.

Buzard KA, Haight D, Troutman R: Ruiz procedure for postkeratoplasty astigmatism. *J Refract Surg*. 1987, 3:40-45.

Nordan LT: Quantifiable astigmatism correction: concepts and suggestions. *J Cataract Refract Surg*. Baltimore, MD. Williams and Wilkins, 1986, 12:507-518.

Percival SPB, Thornton SP: The Plan for Eyes With Ametropia and Astigmatism. In Percival SPB (ed): *A Colour Atlas of Lens Implantation*. St. Louis, MO, Mosby Year Book, 1991.

Chapter 13: Computer Assisted Corneal Topography

Dulaney D, Thornton SP, Martin RG: Corneal Topography in Refractive Surgical Procedures. In Sanders DR, Koch DD (eds):*Corneal Topography*. Thorofare, NJ, SLACK, 1993.

Klyce SD, Wilson SE: Methods of analysis of corneal topography. *Refract Corneal Surg*. Thorofare, NJ. SLACK, 1989, 5:369-371.

Koch DD, Foulks GN, Moran CT, Wakil JS: The EyeSys corneal analysis system: accuracy and reproducibility of first-generation prototype. *Refract Corneal Surg*. Thorofare, NJ. SLACK, 1989, 5:424-429.

Verity SM, Wilson SE, Conger DL: Accuracy and precision of the EyeSys and TMS-1 computerized corneal topographic analysis systems, ARVO abstract. *Invest Ophthalmol Vis Sci*. 1991, 32:1000.

Legeais JM, Ren Q, Simon G, Parel, JM: Computer-assisted corneal topography: accuracy and reproducibility of the topographic modeling system, *Refract Corneal Surg*. Thorofare, NJ. SLACK, 1993, 9:347-357.

Chapter 15: Complications of RK

John ME, Schmidt TE: Traumatic hyphema after radial keratotomy. *Ann Ophthalmol*. 1983: 15(10):930-932.

Neumann AC, Osher RH, Fenzl RE: Radial keratotomy: a clinical and statistical analysis. *Cornea*. 1983, 2:47-55.

Binder P, et al: Delayed wound healing after radial keratotomy. *Am J Ophthalmol*. Chicago, IL. Ophthalmic Publishing, 1985, 92:734-740.

Deitz MR, Sanders DR, Raanan MG: Progressive hyperopia in radial keratotomy: long term follow up of diamond blade and metal blade series. *Ophthalmology*. Philadelphia, PA. J.B. Lippincott, 1986, 93:1284-1289.

O'Day DM, Feman SS, Elliott JH: Visual impairment following radial keratotomy: a cluster of cases. *Ophthalmology*. Philadelphia, PA. J.B. Lippincott, 1986, 93:319-326.

Shivitz IA, Arrowsmith PN: Delayed keratitis after radial keratotomy. *Arch Ophthalmol*. Chicago, IL. American Medical Association, 1986, 104:1153-1155.

Marmer RH: Radial keratotomy complications. *Ann Opthalmol*. 1987, 19:409-411.

Chapter 16: Re-operations

Villasenor R, Cox K: Radial keratotomy: re-operations. *J Refract Surg*. 1:34-37, 1985.

Chen R, Liang Y, Tsai J & Wu F: Surgical results of second attempt radial keratotomy. *Invest Ophthalmol*. 1985, 17:618-620.

Franks S: Radial keratotomy undercorrections: A new approach. *J Refract Surg*. 1986, 2:171-173.

Menezo JL, Cisneros AL, Harto MA: Radial keratotomy: re-operations. *J Refract Surg*. 1988, 4:60-62.

Thornton SP: A comparison of one-stage radial keratotomy with two-stage radial keratotomy. *Refract and Corneal Surg*. Thorofare, NJ. SLACK, Jan 1989, 5:43-45.

Chapter 17: Management of Overcorrection

Waring G, Lynn M, Gelender H, et al: Results of the prospective evaluation of radial keratotomy (PERK) study. *Ophthalmology*. Philadelphia, PA. J.B. Lippincott, 1985, 92:177-198.

Starling JC, Hofmann RF: The new surgical technique for the correction of hyperopia after radial keratotomy: experimental model. *J Refract Surg*. 1986, 2:9-14.

Linquist TD, Williams PA, Lindstrom RL: Management of overcorrection following astigmatic keratotomy. *J Refract Surg*. 1988, 4:218-221.

Index